Redefining Self-Help

Frank Riessman
David Carroll

Redefining
Self-Help

· ·

Policy and Practice

Jossey-Bass Publishers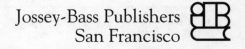
San Francisco

Substantial discounts on bulk quantities of Jossey-Bass books are available to corpora-
tions, professional associations, and other organizations. For details and discount
information, contact the special sales department at Jossey-Bass Inc., Publishers.
(415) 433–1740; Fax (800) 605–2665.

For sales outside the United States, please contact your local Paramount Publishing
International Office.

 Manufactured in the United States of America on Lyons Falls Pathfinder Trade-
book. This paper is acid-free and 100 percent totally chlorine-free.

Library of Congress Cataloging-in-Publication Data

Riessman, Frank, date.
   Redefining self-help : policy and practice / Frank Riessman, David Carroll.
     p.   cm. — (The Jossey-Bass health series)
   Includes bibliographical references and index.
   ISBN 0-7879-0066-4
   1. Self-help groups. I. Carroll, David, date. II. Title. III. Series.
HV547. R55 1995
362.1' 0425—dc20   94-38982
                                                       CIP

FIRST EDITION
HB Printing 10 9 8 7 6 5 4 3 2 1   Code 9523

Contents

Dedicated to Julie Riessman

In 1977, Alan Gartner and I wrote *Self-Help and the Human Services*. Since then enormous changes have taken place within the self-help movement. I believe that we may see even more important developments in the coming period.

Today our need for services far outstrips what our human services systems can provide. Over thirty million Americans have hypertension, eleven million face emotional depression, and at least ten million are addicted to alcohol and six million to drugs. Sexually transmitted diseases have affected fifty-four million, and over one million of them are HIV-positive. And the list goes on. Our present human services systems cannot possibly cope with the vast burden of these and other conditions.

We need an approach for dealing with these mammoth problems—one that will expand our resources without significantly increasing our costs. The self-help paradigm offers just such a perspective. For example, instead of ten million alcoholics in need of help, we can view these people as potential help givers—*a resource rather than a problem*. Instead of focusing on eleven million diabetics in need, we can see segments of this population monitoring themselves individually and coping collectively in groups.

In this book, we will document this turnaround as consumers of mental services—patients—become dispensers of mental health services; students become peer tutors and counselors; women who have lost a breast band together in mutual aid groups to help each other and other mastectomized individuals. Indeed, there are self-help groups for people with every illness identified by the World Health Organization.

When I decided to write *Redefining Self-Help*, I asked David Carroll, an accomplished writer, to assist me because I wanted it to be more than an academic treatise. In this book, we bring up to date earlier discussions of concepts such as self-determination, decommodification, consumer as producer, and the helper therapy principle. In addition, we survey developments that have transformed the study and the practice of self-help over the past two decades.

One major development is the enormous increase in the numbers of professionals directly involved in self-help groups. In California, for example, 83 percent of self-help groups include professionals, who function in a variety of roles. The potential synergy involved in the professional–self-help connection is an extremely important aspect of the expansion of help-giving resources in recent years. Thus, this book is intended for use by professionals and self-helpers, and the relation of these two forces is threaded throughout.

A critical action perspective of the book relates to what I have called the "help paradox," namely the fact that giving help is more beneficial than receiving it. In response to this issue, the focus of this book is restructuring help *to allow everyone the opportunity to play the helper role, and thus to receive the special benefits accruing to that role*.

Overview

Most work on self-help defines the concept as identical to mutual aid. I do not; rather, Chapter One identifies self-help as the crucial, overarching notion and mutual aid as one of its forms. The term *self-help writ large* refers to the broadened redefinition. The concept of addiction is also redefined. Another term that I like is *macro self-help*, to be distinguished from *micro self-help*, which is appropriately concerned with the mechanisms and characteristics of self-help that contribute to its effectiveness. Excellent work in this area has been done by Katz (1993), Levy (1984), Lieberman (1986), and others. By macro self-help I am referring to issues such as the relationship of self-help to social change, the professional–self-help dynamic, the role of the state, and the relevance of self-help with regard to policy issues. Obviously these topics have micro dimensions as well.

Chapter Two looks at the new roles and changing relationships emerging between professionals and self-helpers.

Alcoholics Anonymous, in my view, is the most codified form of self-help and the most powerful example of self-help influencing professional practice; Chapter Three elaborates on these aspects of AA. Chapters Four, Five, and Six are directly related to physical health–, mental health–, and education-related services.

Chapter Seven describes the role of self-help in relation to the expansion of resources, which is a fundamental concern of the book, and outlines the basic shift implicit in the self-help paradigm. By restructuring help, the paradigm reduces the number of dependent helpees and increases the number of independent helpers, whose contribution is further extended since they benefit from playing the helper role.

Chapter Eight looks at social change and interprets the pervasive role that AA has played, surprising in light of its opposition to political activism.

Although the book naturally takes a positive stance toward self-help, Chapter Nine examines the movement's weaknesses, as well as the strengths and weaknesses of professional practice. In essence, self-help suffers from an underestimation of the importance of controlled observation and systematic accountability, key elements in the armor of the professions, which labor under the burdens of detachment and impersonality.

Acknowledgments

In dealing with the professional "privatization of knowledge," I draw on a particularly important book by Charles Derber and colleagues, *Power in the Highest Degree* (Derber, Schwartz, and Magrass, 1990). I have also been influenced greatly by the work of a departed friend, Alvin W. Gouldner.

Four people whose help I want to acknowledge in particular are Audrey Gartner, executive director of the National Self-Help Clearinghouse and coauthor of Chapter Six; Laura Wadenpfuhl, my longtime superb assistant and critic; S. M. Miller, a tireless and helpful adviser; and my wife, Julie Riessman, to whom this book is dedicated, for broadening my understanding of self-help in its various dimensions.

Others deserving thanks include Erik Banks, Barbara Heller, Frances Jemmott, Jossey-Bass for providing two excellent critical reviewers, and Susan Kanaan, who contributed research for Chapter Five.

New York, New York   Frank Riessman
January 1995

The Authors

Frank Riessman has been involved with self-help for more than forty years—in the 1950s and 1960s as a member of the Booker T. Washington Neighborhood Council; in the 1970s as a member of a Westchester County, New York, men's group; and in the 1980s and 1990s as a member of a Parkinson's support group.

He has also facilitated the formation of dozens of self-help groups, assisted in the development of regional clearinghouses, trained large numbers of people in starting self-help groups, and led hundreds of workshops throughout the country.

He has written three books on self-help and numerous professional articles, conducted research on the effectiveness of self-help groups, served on President Carter's Mental Health Commission in the self-help section, and been personally interviewed by hundreds of newspapers and magazines. Perhaps most important, Riessman conceptualized the helper therapy principle (how helping helps the helper) in 1965, based on observations of the processes occurring in these groups. He is also the editor in chief of *Social Policy*, a magazine much concerned with self-help and human service issues and policies.

Riessman has a Ph.D. degree in social psychology, is a licensed psychologist, was formerly chairman of the Department of Psychology at Bard College, and has been a professor of psychology at the Albert Einstein College of Medicine and a professor of sociology at the City University of New York (CUNY) Graduate School and University Center. He is the director of the National Self-Help Clearinghouse at the CUNY Graduate School and University Center.

David Carroll received his B.A. degree from Harvard University. Fifteen of his network TV programs have been produced, including a series of one-man shows for the Public Broadcasting System and the Emmy Award–winning adaptation of *All Quiet on the Western Front* for the *Hallmark Hall of Fame*. Since 1985, he has specialized in books and films on consumer- and patient-oriented medical concerns. His three-part book series (*When Your Loved One Has Alzheimer's*, *Living with Parkinson's Disease*, and *Living Well with MS*) has set standards in the field, and the *Home Medical Handbook, Living with Dying*, and *The Complete Book of Children's Allergies* have all gone into multiple printings. Carroll has written health-related videos and has contributed to pharmaceutical company seminars, reports, and special events for a number of producers. He is devoted to consumer-oriented health education and to making medical topics accessible to the general public.

Redefining Self-Help

What Is Self-Help?

For many years, we have struggled with the term *self-help*. Considering that most of our work relates to mutual aid groups, it has always seemed peculiar to call this activity *self*-help when much of what happens is group behavior.

The theme of self-help has been powerfully emphasized in the history of the black community, from Booker T. Washington to Malcolm X to Jesse Jackson. A few years ago, Benjamin Hooks, former executive director of the National Association for the Advancement of Colored People (NAACP), formed the National Black Organization (NBO), committed to self-help in a communal sense within the African-American community. The emphasis was on the community helping itself, building on its own resources.

Community self-help is indeed widespread, as is reflected in the Community Development Movement and in organizations such as the Bedford Stuyvesant Restoration Corporation in Brooklyn. Grassroots groups have played an important role in revitalizing these neighborhoods.

Self-care has enabled individual diabetics to administer their own insulin (Levin, Katz, and Holtz, 1976, p. 13) and permitted some forty-three million people to quit smoking on their own (rather than in programs such as those conducted by the American Cancer Society; Prochaska and others, 1992; Peele and Brodsky,

1991; Peele, 1989). There are also economic self-help groups, such as food cooperatives, barter groups, and networks such as the Savings Network in Virginia and the Surburban Job Link in Chicago.

The term *self-help* was often used in the early days of the women's movement and the disability rights movement to refer both to mechanisms such as consciousness-raising groups and the Centers for Independent Living and to the underlying philosophy of these movements.

And, of course, the term is widely used in relation to mutual aid groups. Alcoholics Anonymous initially did not use the term *self-help*, but most other twelve-step groups do use it, albeit with some reservations, maintaining that mutual aid is not self-help, meaning individual help.[1]

The media tend to use the term to convey a sense of pulling oneself up by one's bootstraps, in contrast to receiving outside assistance.

A number of what might be called quasi-self-help forms also exist: professionally facilitated support groups, peer helping in schools, tenants becoming public housing managers. These forms use aspects of the self-help approach, with some limitations: the involvement of professionals as trainers and managers of peer groups in schools dilutes the self-help model.

Self-help books make up a huge market. They range from Derek Humphrey's *Last Exit* to books on how to prepare your own income tax return or build your own house. Not necessarily labeled self-help, books such as Bill Wilson's *Alcoholics Anonymous*, Betty Friedan's *Feminine Mystique*, and Melanie Beatty's books on codependency nevertheless all conform to a similar model, in somewhat greater depth. Self-help books and tapes remain on the margin, as they are mostly the marketed products of writers, experts, and professionals; nonetheless, they do provide considerable personal empowerment, including consumer choice, and respond to the implicit demands of people for involvement in their own betterment.

The Internal Versus the External

What, then, do all these self-help examples have in common? They seem to contrast sharply with external interventions by teachers, experts, the clergy, group therapists, or the state. Sometimes *internal self-help* intervention is in opposition to the more frequently prescribed external approach; at other times the relationship is more subtle.

Most important is that both approaches share the basic self-help philosophy, an emphasis on promoting latent inner strengths, and the special understanding that comes from proximity to the problem or need. Essential to this conceptualization is the emphasis on self-determination, self-reliance, self-production, and self-empowerment—all stressing the internal resources, whether in relation to the production of services or help or of governance and power.

Moreover, self-help is not synonymous with individual help, though sometimes it may be exactly that. If we look at the examples cited, self-help emphasizes internal resources in contradistinction to a variety of other approaches, all of which emphasize external intervention, help coming from the outside, from church or state or professional expert.[2]

The problem becomes confusing because sometimes the internal self-help unit is a group or a community and sometimes it is an individual, as in giving up smoking or using a self-help book. So there is such a thing as individual self-help, but there is also nonindividual self-help.

Indeed, the self-help unit can be an individual, a group (even such broad ones as women, the disabled, or gay people), a community, and even the entire nation. Thus the self-help of individuals who quit smoking on their own can be contrasted with antismoking programs of the American Cancer Society; the self-help mutual aid of alcoholics participating in AA can be contrasted with traditional approaches that emphasize willpower and view alcoholism as a moral issue (the latter approach is very different from the philosophy developed by alcoholics themselves); and the self-help orientation of African Americans, concerned with using and developing the internal resources of their community, can be contrasted with the external interventions proposed by the government or experts outside the community.

This redefinition of self-help may be satisfying in one sense because of its parsimonious, coherent integration of the relevant phenomena. But what difference does it make? What are the consequences of this reformulation? It underscores the importance of the essence of self-help, which is not mutual aid but rather an emphasis on the internal resources and potential strengths of the self-help unit (individual, group, or community).[3] In this sense, self-help thinking merges with the whole body of knowledge regarding regeneration in the health sphere, which emphasizes the body's self-healing propensities and judges external forces on their facilitating or deterrent effects.

The important distinction here is between healing and curing: "The term healing [is used] to refer to what is done *by* the patient (or the patient's body) in order to resolve a problem of the body, mind, or spirit; whereas the term curing usually refers to what is done to the patient by a physician or therapist" (Upledger, 1989, p. 67).

The Self-Help Paradigm

The reconceptualization of the self-help paradigm views people with problems as potential help givers, as more independent than dependent. The paradigm changers the helper/helpee ratio in numerous ways:

1. The number of individuals involved exclusively in helpee roles is vastly reduced, and the number of helpers is increased dramatically.

2. Even when receiving help the receiver knows that tomorrow or even later at the same meeting he or she will provide help

to someone else, which removes the loss of status experienced by one who is only a helpee.

3. The help-giving power of the entire unit is expanded because of the power that emanates from so many individuals playing the helping role.

Resources for help increase not only quantitatively but qualitatively as well, because the new helping behavior in the system derives from the experience of the help seekers, the people with the problem, whose latent potential has previously been passive but is now activated. Also, the entire process of giving and receiving help has been democratized and shared, further contributing to the qualitative change. A new ethos has been born.

On the one hand, the paradigm is a vision; on the other, it is a tool providing a methodology for seeing problems in a nonpathological way; it releases energy that change agents can then activate.

The Self-Help Ethos

Perhaps the best way to understand the essence of self-help is through an examination of the self-help ethos, especially its emphasis on empowerment and a bottom-up orientation, as well as a number of other features. The strength of the self-help movement, indeed, lies not in its structure or organization but in its spirit and worldview, as embodied in the self-help ethos. Because of its significance, it may be useful here to elaborate on its various dimensions.

The self-help ethos is a constellation of norms and sentiments, a series of themes that underlie behavior. It is a unique configuration that includes both old and new traditions. It is essentially an "ideal type" construction: no self-help entity exhibits all its possible characteristics or dimensions. And other consumer movements—neighborhood, disability rights—embody many of the same characteristics, which, incidentally, may serve as a possible basis for the development of interconnections to these movements and their mutual strengthening. The ethos transcends individual groups and reduces the fragmentation inherent in a self-help movement that takes so many different forms.

Oppositional Themes

One of the dimensions of this ethos, the "anti-big" dimension, reflects a response to problems inherent in modern society as related to scale, bureaucracy, and impersonality. Bureaucratic organization is characterized by hierarchy, impersonal rules, and a division of labor that emphasizes technical competence. Self-help, by contrast, is highly personal; competence is based on experience, it does not have a highly differentiated division of labor, and it is typically nonhierarchical.

Although bureaucracy may have some relevance when dealing with large-scale problems, a dialectic balance is needed to limit the problems brought about by its size. The self-help ethos provides a response to this problem by emphasizing the personal, the informal, the simple, the direct. It works through member understanding and networking rather than organizational control from the top. Moreover, the self-help experience develops competencies and skills to help people cope more effectively with bureaucratic structures and to develop nonbureaucratic ways of dealing with large-scale problems.

A second major theme in this regard is directed toward a reaffirmation of basic core traditions as related to the role of community, neighborhood, spiritual values, and self-reliance. Implicit in this theme is a cry against certain aspects of modernism, combining as it does a reaffirmation of old populist traditions with a strong antagonism toward hedonism, corruption, drugs, and violence, all of which are perceived as being related to the breakdown of social norms and positive traditions.

These two themes are, in a sense, "antithemes." But typical of the self-help way, they take the form of a selective acknowledgment and acceptance of the old, together with support for new approaches that constrain the negative consequences of modern organization.

Empowerment and Participation

To some extent, the empowerment theme implicit in self-help reflects aspects of modern life yet also carries forward the participatory mode of earlier decades. The new element is the strong accent on exerting control over one's life. One aspect of this motif is a reaction to the sense of powerlessness that people feel with regard to major issues over which they have no control—the economy, world peace, social pathology—but other sources of this empowerment relate to vast increases in both formal and informal education and an expanded consumer role. The participatory theme is reflected in networking, shared leadership, peer processes, mutual aid, and what Toffler calls the *prosumer*—the consumer as producer of services (Toffler, 1980).

New Age Psychology

Another promodern theme implicit in self-help relates to self-acceptance and openness and encompasses an attitude of opposition toward the forces in society that portray differentness negatively. I'm OK, you're OK, everyone is OK: women, gays, the disabled, stutterers, victims of abuse, little people, minorities, old people, the homeless, fat people, and, if they accept the problem, even victimizers of others (Parents Anonymous, Batterers Anonymous) and self-victimizers (gamblers, drug addicts, sexaholics). This theme represents a significant breakthrough in human relations, releasing enormous energy and reframing self-images.

The Democratization of Everyday Life

The democratic theme in the self-help ethos is powerful and central to the entire self-help constellation. It puts democratic values to work in important new ways, extending the meaning of democracy at the personal level and in the private domain. It also reenergizes traditional democratic concepts relating to the participation theme.

Demystification is another element of the democratic theme. People have the right to know. Jargon and circuitous explanations are anathema; simple, direct principles are preferred.

Antielitism and antiexpertism are also significant. The accent here is on experience-based wisdom and on understanding from the perspective of the insider. The people who have the problem are part of the solution.

In a very important way, the self-help approach represents an extension of the worldwide movement toward democracy. The democracy movement is primarily concerned with issues of governance, while self-help philosophy extends the involvement of consumers beyond the decision-making role to the production of help and services. Also relevant is the democratization of everyday life, in particular, the destigmatization of all kinds of behavior, including mental illness and physical disability. Perhaps no group is more open to expanded participation than the massive numbers of chronically ill people whose participation in their own care is a critical health component. The significance of the phrase "I alone can change my condition, but I cannot do it alone" underlies the importance of individual power to the collective.

Reconceptualizing Addiction

Nowhere is the self-help ethos more evident than in its opposition to addiction. In fact, one way to understand the essence of self-help is to see it as a contrasting, countervailing force to addiction.

We formulate the concept of addiction in two ways, described as simple addiction and complex addiction, each with different implications for action or intervention. Simple addiction applies to any substance or process that produces a powerful physical dependency, a craving, and a strong withdrawal reaction. A patient in a hospital receiving morphine to control pain may fall prey to simple addiction. But it is generally not difficult to wean the individual from the drug, reducing the withdrawal effects over a relatively short period of time.

In complex addiction, the substance or process takes on deeper meaning in relation to the individual's character structure. Moreover, the addictive behavior is highly resistant to change and rationality and becomes part of a larger compulsive pattern of behavior.

Research indicates that there are four central elements to complex addiction (Du Pont and McGovern, 1994; Schaef and Fassel, 1988; Carnes 1983). The first is that the addictive behavior produces good feelings or eliminates bad feelings (or both). The second is loss of control over the addictive behavior. Third, the addictive behavior persists despite problems that it causes. The fourth central element is denial.

Complex addiction occurs when a substance or process is used to alter a mood—that is, when something external is employed to affect an internal state, not requiring any inner work or self-help.[4]

In our view, complex addiction is far more significant than simple addiction. Let us illustrate with the case of nicotine. The fact that millions of people have quit smoking on their own is evidence that their behavior, while reflecting a particularly powerful physical dependency (simple addiction), can nevertheless be altered.

We hypothesize that there are two kinds of cigarette smokers. For one type, smoking has deep addictive meaning (it is a complex addiction), and they cannot shake the habit. The other group is similar to individuals who have acquired a powerful physical dependency in their hospital use of morphine and are able to surrender the habit with varying degrees of effort because it lacks deep meaning and power (Glassman, 1993).

We suspect that there are also two types of drinkers (apart from the traditionally defined typology of alpha, beta, gamma, and delta). One type is the drinker with a complex addiction who requires an intensive program such as Alcoholics Anonymous or a professional rehabilitative program. The assumption here is that altering this behavior, which is deeply rooted and probably affected by the biological makeup of the individual, requires a strong intervention and a long period of recovery. This intervention attempts to provide addicted individuals with a new spiritual philosophy and a well-developed support system, both aimed at achieving sobriety.

There are probably a number of individuals who may acquire a strong physical dependency on drinking (simple addiction to alcohol) but may be able to change this behavior without recourse to the AA model. They may be quite receptive to traditional habit-breaking techniques. Some of these individuals may even be able to acquire the habit of controlled drinking.[5]

Let us illustrate with an example from personal experience. For over thirty years Frank Riessman had two large martinis every evening before dinner. These drinks were very important to him, so important that his family and friends often thought he might be an alcoholic. Yet upon learning that he had diabetes, he stopped drinking immediately and experienced no withdrawal symptoms whatsoever. He has not had a drink again for over four years. However, despite his intimate knowledge of the deleterious effects of sweets on diabetics, he has been unable to shake a complex addiction to ice cream and cake despite repeated efforts, and even small attempts at abstinence cause considerable depression and anxiety.

In essence, the self-help worldview is totally antithetical to complex addiction, which is, of course, the significant addiction in our society. The self-help approach looks inward for understanding and for the development of coping responses to problems. Its inward look can be to the individual, the mutual aid group, or the community. The addictive model seeks an answer from outside and is primarily concerned with compulsive alteration of the mood or state that accompanies a problem; in other words, it is concerned with a surface dimension, temporarily reducing tension but never solving the problem.

Detoxification and traditional behavior modification are never sufficient for individuals with complex addiction, and relapse is common. These people have no choice but to abstain from the addictive substance, as it will reactivate the addictive pattern.

People actually afflicted with an addiction, moreover, represent only the tip of the iceberg. Their pathology expresses, in extreme form, the underlying addictive tendency that is so pervasive in our consumer society (Schaef, 1987; Forbes, 1994). The negative side of modern consumerism—the side that gives rise to the abnormality of addiction—forces the consumer to select quick approaches to external objects and processes available in the marketplace. This process is accentuated and highlighted by the media. We are encouraged, even cajoled, to buy something for every discomfort, every problem—right now!

There is even an effort afoot to "sell" self-help groups in the same fashion. This has led to something of a backlash, as critics decry the zealous hyping of recovered addicts on the popular talk shows, most of whom promote self-help in a highly distorted way. The problem is that we cannot buy self-help; it is not a commodity but rather something that the consumer has to produce, essentially from the inner resources and (codified) experience of the individual, mutual aid group, community, or oppressed group.

The millions of drug addicts, compulsive eaters, gamblers, and debtors are all on the same continuum as the normal person. This is what Erich Fromm (1947) dubbed the "pathology of normalcy," pointing out that the pathology highlights the basic tendencies of the society. We are not suggesting a lack of qualitative difference between the drug addict and the rest of us. Addiction requires new methods of intervention. Above all, the addict needs other addicts as a necessary component for recovery—people who understand from the inside, from direct experience, who have followed a path that promises some degree of control for the illness.

The reason why we argue in Chapter Eight that the self-help movement is such a critical factor for deep social change is not just that its methods appear to have a broad impact on the pathology but also that its worldview opposes the prevailing narcissistic compulsive consumerism.[6] Indeed, its ideological premises are neither radical nor conservative nor liberal, though it draws on all of these as it goes head to head with commercialism, the money culture that pervades every corner of our society (including professional use of portions of the self-help apparatus in the form of rehabilitation and recovery). The self-help motif draws on the best in the tradition of religion, especially its spiritual features, emphasizing the values of cooperation, caring, transformation, and community.

How did the self-help worldview come about? It would be easy to answer that it emerged from pain, and at a certain level this is valid. But that response is incomplete. We believe that the self-help worldview derives from other dimensions of the consumer role, a role that contains the seeds of empowerment. After all, consumers are critically needed to make the system work, to use and buy the products and services that have resulted from the tremendous productivity of advanced capitalism and, at a simpler level, to provide the stimulus to move the business cycle. It is no accident that the major movements of our time have come from individuals functioning in their consumer roles—women, neighborhood residents, free speech students, and so on (Gartner and Riessman, 1974).

The positive consumerist dimensions focus heavily on the power of choice and potential empowerment and lead ultimately to the desire to make a difference. The self-help movement is a product of this free space that has not been turned into a commodity or a bureaucracy.

The essence of self-help lies in a philosophy that emphasizes the potential inner strength of the individual, the group, the community. Self-help thus means help built around the inner core and is typically contrasted with help offered from the outside, along with the more traditional mainstream forms of assistance.

"Self-help writ large" is meant to include all the various forms of self-help and all the quasi-self-help entities. This approach gives the concept much greater breadth and significance than, say, self-help mutual aid groups alone. It attempts to show the link among the many forms of self-help, all of which reflect the philosophy.[7]

A Bit of History

Before the advent of Alcoholics Anonymous, self-help often came through the friendly societies, consumer cooperatives, and ethnic-based groups of early-twentieth-century America. The friendly societies developed to help people cope with the stresses of industrialization. They not only dealt with the immediate needs of their members but also served to politicize them (Katz and Bender, 1976). In the United States, one response to the industrial revolution in the nineteenth century was to create utopian cooperative villages or communes, such as the Owenite society. Large-scale immigration to America led to the formation of various mutual benefit societies, including free-loan societies and burial societies.

The formation of Alcoholics Anonymous in 1935 began the modern era of self-help. AA developed a twelve-step model emulated today by over one hundred other groups, such as Gamblers Anonymous, Overeaters Anonymous, and Debtors Anonymous. Although AA, as an organization, is opposed to political action, it does not discourage individual members from such involvement. (The impact of AA on institutional change is discussed in Chapter Eight.)

In the late 1960s and the 1970s, the women's movement also played a pivotal role in promoting self-help advocacy. The basic unit was the small consciousness-raising group, which was initially concerned with issues of identity. Self-help characterized many of the practices of these groups. This modality was extended into the women's health movement (*Our Bodies, Ourselves*, by the Boston Women's Health Book Collective, 1946), and then to large-scale

social and political issues. Together with the disability rights movement and the gay rights movement, the women's movement provides an important model for present-day self-help advocacy as is
now expressed in a large number of advocacy-oriented self-help
groups: the National Alliance for the Mentally Ill (NAMI), Mothers Against Drunk Driving (MADD), Self-Help for the Hard of
Hearing, Victims for Victims, and so on.

In 1978, President Carter's Mental Health Commission proposed the self-help approach as a major mental health intervention.
Among its specific proposals was the development of self-help clearinghouses and self-help directories. In 1979, the National Self-Help
Clearinghouse was organized, and in the ensuing decade, more than
sixty regional and local clearinghouses arose. These clearinghouses
provide information and referral, training, research, and public education and continue to play an important role in relating professionals to self-help groups. By holding conferences and fairs, the
clearinghouses bring together a large number of separate self-help
groups, enabling them to establish a common identity and ethos.

On the basis of two surveys using large household samples, an
estimated 7.5 million adults participated in a self-help mutual aid
group in 1992 (Lieberman and Snowden, 1993). The most rapidly
growing segments of the self-help movement appear to be twelve-
step groups modeled after AA, advocacy-oriented groups such as
MADD, and disabled rights groups, which have had a dramatic
impact on national legislation. Since the 1960s, the self-help
approach has also been utilized in the neighborhood movement and
in community action.

While our presentation of the history of self-help focuses essentially on the mutual aid group form, it should be noted that the various other forms of self-help, such as peer helping, books and tapes,
and professionally facilitated support groups, more or less came into
their own in the period from the late 1970s to the present.

It is often argued with considerable merit that self-help mutual
aid has been less than fully responsive to people of color, but this
argument appears to be less accurate when considering such forms

of self-help as peer helping in the schools, community action and economic self-help groups, consumer-managed mental health centers, and tenant-managed public housing. It is also notable that in the past decade, AA has moved sharply away from its white male predominance to include large numbers of women and people of color.

As one examines the landscape of behaviors and forms that are sometimes envisioned as self-help (such as gangs, the Nation of Islam, and other severely nationalistic expressions), it becomes clear that the concept is open to broad interpretation. Although much of the self-help ethos is highly participatory and deeply extends democratic values, it is not consistently progressive. Excessively nationalistic internal biases appear to arise from long-term rejection by major external forces. In a defensive reaction, the internal unit totally opposes all external assistance with a weird intensity.

In the process of development, a strong internal emphasis is a natural first-step as the self-help unit gathers its resources, building strengths that then permit a more selective interaction with the external forces. Prime examples of this are seen in the women's and disabled-people's rights movements. We are not referring here only to the utilization of self-help forms, such as consciousness-raising groups among women, in the early stages of these movements, but rather to the self-help dimension that goes far beyond this expression and is much more related to the building on and building up of inner resources.

Why Now?

Crowded out in the 1960s by social movements such as civil rights, Vietnam, free speech, and the counterculture, the self-help movement began to pick up large numbers of adherents in the 1970s, then hit its full stride a decade later in the Reagan-Bush era.

At present, a self-help group is available for every major disorder listed by the World Health Organization. Some groups exist for diseases so rare that many doctors have never heard of them.

Self-help groups exist for procrastinators, overeaters, overspenders, burn victims, prostitutes, sexaholics, workaholics, amputees, and parents who abuse their children; for the hearing impaired, the blind, and the spouses of chronic snorers; for drug addicts of every kind and degree; for Holocaust survivors; for sufferers of incest trauma; for bereaved parents, grandparents raising grandchildren, and parents without partners.

All the members of these groups are, of course, pioneers by dint of the fact that they are taking the bull by the horns and creating a group support situation where none existed before. They are also breaking fresh ground in a more subtle way, by circumventing hospitals and lawyers' offices and political rallies and psychology clinics and seeking help instead in communal and community-based nonprofessional arenas. For them, "legitimacy is not conferred by professionals but decided on by the consumers of services" (Katz, 1993, p. 80).

All these people are common victims of the social woes typical of life in the 1990s. We all know the list: destruction of the environment; an inefficient medical care system; loss of a sense of belonging, of personal belief and shared moral values. Add to this the growing skepticism toward political authority, everyday fears of unchecked crime and rampant substance abuse, deterioration of our schools, the breakup of the nuclear family, and the pitting of race against race, young against old, male against female, husband against wife, rich against poor, parent against child. On top of this pile the drudgery of automated labor, alienation at the workplace, and the divorce between production and pride of workmanship. Even the computer, with its reputed ability to streamline office chores, ultimately hobbles as much as it helps, generating more paper than ever before, causing companywide delays when the main machine "goes down," and making users feel like robots in an updated office version of *Modern Times*.

Alongside these global imbroglios are more local and personal ones. The American neighborhood, so long a bulwark against isolation, even in big cities, has been transformed from a community of mutually helping neighbors into a beehive of hermetically sealed cells. In many urban areas, apartment dwellers go decades without knowing the name or even the face of the person living next door. Even in small towns, a new concern with crime and safety now causes people to build fences and double-lock their doors.

The decline of neighborhoods, increased mobility, and the breakdown of family relationships have all contributed to the emergence of self-help mutual aid groups, sometimes called the "new neighborhoods." People are looking for connections, for community, and for ways to reduce their isolation. Many decry the loss of community and the rise of rampant individualism in American life. The self-help movement is one important response to this condition. Wuthnow's study (*Sharing the Journey: Support Groups and America's New Quest for Community,* 1994) provides further support for the thesis that people are looking for community and finding it in a huge number of support groups, particularly small Bible study groups.

Also hurt are those in need: the poor, the homeless, the bankrupt, the disenfranchised. Society has consistently failed to supply these millions with an equal distribution of professional helping services; and when these services do in fact arrive, they are often served up in such bureaucratic and punitive ways that recipients feel more like victims than the receivers of nurturant aid. Searching for options, they often discover that self-help represents a no-cost alternative to professional services.

In sum, many of the communal supports that once gave our forbears a sense of group solidarity have disappeared from modern life, leaving us without anchor or sense of tribe. In their place are substituted the cold comforts of competition, rampant individualism, bureaucracy, the TV set, and the prying eye of the technostate. How ironic that in a country founded on the principles of independence and autonomy, a majority of people now find their sense of self-determination inhibited, Gulliver-like, by a vast web of intersecting societal cords—not just the heavy ropes of national problems and government strictures but the petty strings of the credit check and the permit bureau, the tax audit and the lost insurance form, plus the thousand and one laws promulgated by a legal system that often seems more interested in controlling its citizens than improving their lives.

What is the result of all these frustrations and trammels? Simply this: that more and more people in our society feel like expendable pawns. The loneliness and anomie created by this condition ultimately add up to a string of inescapable perplexities and neglects for a majority of ordinary people that are soon transformed into a regimen of lacks: lack of effectiveness and influence, lack of caring human contact, lack of purpose or meaning in life, lack of personal control.

Herein lie the critical reasons for the empowerment movement.

Sources of the Quest for Empowerment

It would be easy to say that the demand for empowerment arises because people have been disempowered and feel that lack. However, demands do not simply arise from needs. Revolutions typically do not occur at the lowest point but rather when expectations are rising in light of changing conditions and new possibilities. The civil rights movement emerged in the 1960s in a period of economic expansion, in the aftermath of World War II, when blacks served in the armed forces and worked in the factories. New expectations arose from that experience.

What new conditions have emerged to give rise to the quest for empowerment, the desire to increase control over one's life? Some immediate factors and some deep underlying roots can be identified.

1. A long-range underlying cause is related to the significance of the consumer role in an advanced capitalist society. Consumers

are needed to absorb the goods resulting from vastly expanded productive capacity. Selling and advertising become central enterprises
directed at the consumer. And although it is conventional to
emphasize the exploitation and manipulation of the consumer, there
is another side that is to some extent taken for granted and under-
stated—the fact that the consumer has choices. They may be limited choices, but the consumer is nevertheless involved in
appraising, questioning, choosing, and evaluating. Out of this
choosing process, the consumer develops the beginnings of feelings
of power (perhaps sometimes exaggerated), plus various skills in
making choices. Consumerism and the consumer movement arise
as a way of strengthening the consumers in their choices (and prac-
tically all of the movements of the past twenty-five years have been
consumer-based and built around consumer issues—rents, crime,
human services). This choosing dimension is the forerunner of the
empowerment orientation. Obviously, empowerment is more than
choosing in the marketplace and more than the power of choice
alone. But the underlying feeling and the skills associated with
choosing form an important base that, together with other dimensions, serves to stimulate increased empowerment.

2. In our society, most services, such as health, education, and
mental health, frequently involve the consumer closely with the
seller and sometimes with service production itself. For example,
consumers do their own shopping in the supermarket, fill out their
own deposit slips in banks, and participate closely in their own
health practice. The human services are particularly consumer-
intensive: the consumer potentially contributes to the productivity
of the service. This process might even be far better developed were
it not for the ambivalence of the providers of the service. Nevertheless, consumer power does expand the feelings of choice, control, and involvement and perhaps nurtures the wish for more.

3. The tremendous expansion of education, both formal and
informal, is also critical to the appeal of empowerment. Education

has grown tremendously in the past twenty years as far greater numbers of students graduate from high schools and colleges. Perhaps even more important is the enormous expansion of informal education arising from the media, particularly television. Whatever the limitations of the media, they impart information, verbal skills, and models and do so in a pervasive, entertaining fashion. Education is particularly empowering. It can increase the desire for control over one's own life.

4. Major political events in the past two decades have contributed to a decline in respect for authority and experts and an increase in respect for experiential knowledge. Watergate and Vietnam were instrumental in the debunking of big authority. The free speech, student, and new left movements of the 1960s were also contributing factors. Investigative journalism and the media's interest in muckraking also play a role.

Trust in big institutions—government, the professions, business—is likewise in decline. Distrust of big power dovetails with increased respect for the layperson, for experience, for peers. All of this is expressed in the self-help movement with its populist anti-expertism, critique of professionalism, and concomitant respect for the average person.

Another aspect of this distrust is expressed both in individual and collective forms, in the women's movement; in books such as *Our Bodies, Ourselves,* which sold over four million copies in its first edition; in the women's health movement; in consciousness-raising groups; and ultimately in more advanced political forms.

Underlying all these themes is the fact that the majority of people in our society have not felt able to cope with, or even to understand, large issues related to foreign policy or national economic policy. People feel a lack of control in these matters and are mystified by the processes involved. For the most part, they have retreated from this larger agenda and have moved their demands for empowerment to local issues and narrower interest group questions.

As people gain strength, experience, and competence in these local issues, to some extent they move back to the larger agenda.

What Makes Self-Help Work?

Most people feel that they cannot make the economy better or reduce the national debt. They know that they cannot repair the ozone hole or make peace in the Middle East. These things are too big, too abstract, too far away.

What can individuals do to take back their lost sense of power? For starters, they can move from the hopelessly huge canvas of world affairs down to a smaller, more manageable medium where individual influence once again becomes an option: to their neighborhood, their families, their private lives. Here they find the sense of control denied them on the global level. Here they really can do something to help an aging parent or to overcome an eating addiction. They can set wheels in motion when the city won't fix the streetlights on their block or if they want to talk to others about being gay.

The people who look to the smaller picture, moreover, achieve empowerment without relying on entrenched establishment authorities for help. How? By relying instead on local resources—specifically, on other people with the same problems as themselves, people who congregate on a regular basis at a particular locale with the express purpose of solving a specific life problem and of gaining back at least part of the power that's been taken from them.

In this sense, self-help represents not a rebellion against the imperial giantism of the modern world but rather a return to the more governable limits of neighborhood, friends, family, and self. In a world where problems are expanding, resources are thinning, expert solutions are wanting, and the voice of the individual is lost in the crowd, the friendly self-help group meeting around the corner seems just the place to take back one's lost sense of power, self-value, and control.

What specific features of self-help make it so attractive to contemporary Americans and so enlivening for its adherents? The following aspects—to which we shall return at various times throughout the book—serve as a working basis.

Transformation of Needs into Assets

First and in many ways foremost, the self-help movement allows people to convert their needs and problems into assets. Running head on into an encounter with dependency, sickness, or addiction, people who pass through this needle's eye emerge with firsthand knowledge of how their problem works and what can be done to cope with it.

Such individuals become, as it were, living resources and are ideally positioned to convert their knowledge into a potent force for guiding—and changing—other people who suffer from similar difficulties. In this way, the problem becomes part of the solution.

In this sense, members of Gamblers Anonymous or Overeaters Anonymous are not simply suffering addicts. They are experts on the subject of addiction, and this makes them singularly qualified to counsel others with a similar affliction.

Interchangeability of Roles

Recently, as part of a comprehensive districtwide peer-tutoring program in New York City, a group of eighth graders was recruited to tutor low-achieving seventh graders. The tutors volunteered with great enthusiasm and accepted their rigorous training eagerly, looking forward to working with the "clients," as they called their prospective tutees. There was only one problem: no one volunteered to be a tutee.

The reason, it turned out, was that the already low self-esteem of the potential tutees would have been exacerbated by being singled out to receive help from youngsters their own age who were apparently smarter and better adjusted than themselves. The painful reality for these poor students was that getting help also meant getting hurt.

This strange paradox produces a particularly problematic situation when helper and helpee meet: well aware of the strings and stigmas attached to the help receiver's role, helpees often develop a deep ambivalence toward the helping process itself. Persons may desperately need, even desire, help of some kind. Often, however, they have mixed feelings about the quality of the help they receive, the way in which the help is given, the person who is giving the help, and the fact that they are in this powerless position in the first place.

In the ideal self-help environment, this problem is transcended in several ways. One is by making the roles of helper and helpee interchangeable, that is, by giving all members a chance both to give advice and to receive it, according to the needs of the situation. Another is by distributing authority equally among the membership, thus doing away with a ruling elite and the dominator-dominated interplay that results from both.

Tonight, for example, a member has a problem. I respond with advice. I thus become the expert; the power is mine. Tomorrow night it is I who have a problem, and this same member advises me. Because I gave help last night, the part of my personality that seeks control is pacified, and now I am content to play the role of recipient without feeling inadequate or singled out.

This interchangeability of roles allows members to give and take in equal measure and at the same time reduces the dangers inherent in charismatic, single-person leadership. It is indeed one of AA's most ingenious contributions to have encouraged a shared or circulating leadership among its members, thereby avoiding the power struggles that seem inevitably to undermine every group endeavor.

Positive Ethos

The self-help ethos, or spirit, has a special human dimension to it that people respond to and return to. The atmosphere at mutual aid meetings is generally noncompetitive and cooperative. No one is pitted against anyone; indeed, the success of the group rises or falls on the cooperation of its individual members. At the same time, honesty is valued, and people are encouraged not to pull their punches.

The self-help movement is antipressure and antibureaucratic, fostering a "do what you can" and "one day at a time" philosophy. The general tone is upbeat, can-do, optimistic, with an emphasis on recovery and on one's ability to change for the better. People like this. It helps them view their problems, even the large ones, as solvable and manageable, in some cases even as assets, as potential raw material for achieving the kind of clarity and self-knowledge they might never have known had life not foisted these troubles upon them. It gives them hope.

The self-help approach itself, moreover, is adaptable to a wide range of constituencies, including women, youth, the aged, the sick, and the physically handicapped. Finally, the sense of belonging to something larger and greater than oneself creates a special mystique among the group membership that is in many ways part of the therapeutic process itself.

Self-Help from Inside Experience

Self-help and mutual help groups develop, as it were, from the inside. This means that self-helpers turn to their own experience for models rather than to the conventional wisdom of outside professionals or experts.

The result of this orientation is that self-help is based on an experiential model rather than a theoretical one, on the accumulated knowledge of people who have lived through the very troubles and problems that they are gathered to solve.

This quality of inside orientation extends to the logistics of running the group. Most groups make it a matter of principle to be self-sustaining, to be dependent on their own resources for material needs such as housing and money. Taking the populist model of nonaffiliation and free admission as a basis, political alignments of any kind are avoided, and fundraising is confined to within the group itself. This approach helps make the self-help community a contained unit, one that is dependent on its own resources for growth and sustenance. This fact in turn reinforces a member's basic sense of independence and control.

Accent on Empowerment

The thrust of a self-help or mutual aid group is action, dispatch, effort, responsibility, endeavor, and solving a problem rather than accepting it as a helpless sufferer. Whether or not a person succeeds at this task—and in many cases a partial or even incremental improvement is counted as a victory—the very fact that members have taken an active rather than a passive stance becomes an enlivening and even rehabilitative experience.

In this broadest of senses, the self-help medium is also the self-help message. And that message is empowerment.

Being Helped by Helping

The act of giving help to others is by no means a selfless activity; indeed, it is largely a self-serving one. Talk to group members about the increased confidence and self-esteem that come from guiding other people. Helping, in general, feels good.

Best of the Old and the New

Much about self-help is traditional and comfortable. Besides the emphasis on family and community, its democratic forum harks back to the village meeting or, further, to the tribal council, and its encouragement of caring and service has overtones of age-old traditions.

At the same time, self-help is a child of the late twentieth century. The modern emphasis on mutual self-revelation, sharing, and honesty comes closer, perhaps, to the New Age than to the church or even to Sigmund Freud. So do the concepts of a nonpolitical, self-sustaining, nonaffiliated collectivity, plus the ideas of recovery and removal of self-blame. One of the features that makes self-help so appealing, in short, is that it fuses the old and the new into a synthesis for modern times.

All things considered, then, it is apparent that a new help paradigm has arisen in this country over the past three decades and that this new model is rapidly working its way into the popular consciousness. Members of the self-help movement are no longer patients or clients or consumers of services. They are prosumers, the people who both manufacture the goods (help) and consume them (also help) at the same time.

Under this new paradigm, we no longer think of ten million recovering drug addicts as ten million sick men and women in need of pity and therapeutic assistance. We look at them now as an army of potential teachers and role models who understand drugs better than anyone else in the world. In other words, we see them in a transformed way: as participants in a powerful new conversion process whereby the takers also become the givers and wherein the producers are also the consumers.

This model opens up many new possibilities. Once set in place, for example, it increases the number of available help givers exponentially. By extension, it also reduces the number of dependent helpees.

This paradigm likewise improves the value of help. Active members of a mutual aid group are not simply scholars or licensed practitioners. They are seasoned veterans of the addiction wars, credentialed at the college of real life. This fact ups their credibility as role models and mentors and gives solid authority to their opinions and advice.

Backing them up is a fresh new lexicon of therapeutic principles, ideas born of practical knowledge rather than the observations of others, ideas that have evolved from the sweat and tears of thousands of self-helpers in hundreds of thousands of hours of meetings over the years—ideas such as reciprocity, sharing, interchangeability of roles, a horizontal rather than hierarchic power structure—ideas that make self-help groups tick.

Self-help groups work well for many reasons, including emotional support, shared experience, disclosure, learning of coping skills, normalization, installation of hope, cognitive restructuring, empathy, feedback, reflection, modeling, behavioral prescription, and self-actualization (see Katz, 1993, pp. 33–41; Wollert and others, 1982; Stewart, 1990; Lieberman and Borman, 1991; and Borkman, 1976).

Conclusion

A major reason for the current resonance of the self-help approach relates to the significant world problems to which a self-help model is potentially responsive, including widespread feelings of powerlessness and alienation (for instance, among burned-out human service workers) and of isolation; widespread addictions; the spiritual gap; the tremendous expansion of chronic illnesses; the need for support systems; the help paradox (people in need having problems in receiving help); the professional contradiction, or service versus money; problems associated with bureaucracy and size; the limits of resources; the limits of experts; the rampant greed and corruption; the education crisis; the need for cost-effective approaches that have multiple benefits; the search for a new politics. The potential power of the self-help intervention stems from many sources: the paradigm, the basic principles (self-determination, consumers as producers, helper therapy), the ethos, the expansion of resources, empowerment, the restructuring of help, a sense of community, and the various mechanisms of the mutual aid group that characterize its effectiveness—sharing and disclosure. Its power also derives in large part from the fact that self-help is not a commodity bought and sold in the marketplace. This freedom is what allows the self-help movement its wholeheartedness and commitment.

2

The Professional–Self-Help Dialectic

A major development in the self-help world is the much greater involvement of professionals in self-help groups, in roles ranging from leadership and coleadership to membership. In California, 83 percent of the mutual support groups had professional involvement, in thirteen different roles, some as little as two hours per month and some as much as ten hours (Goodman and Jacobs, 1994). Informal reports from various self-help clearinghouses around the nation support the generalization of new levels of professional involvement.

The situation with regard to twelve-step groups is manifestly different, as professionals qua professionals are permitted no role. Although there was, surprisingly, a low degree of professional involvement in twelve-step groups (Goodman and Jacobs, 1994), the rehabilitation industry and the recovery therapy movement both are composed, as we shall see in Chapter Three, of large numbers of professionals, albeit professionals who are also recovering alcoholics or addicts. And the industry is beholden to twelve-step philosophy and practice in numerous ways, including referrals to Alcoholics Anonymous and AA meetings on rehabilitation sites, treatment, and methodology.

Thus it can be said that both the twelve-step and the non-twelve-step segments of the self-help movement are being deeply affected by professionals.

What are the implications of this? Does it affect the purity of the self-help movement or simply provide more combinations to an already varied population? Before answering these questions, it will be useful to review the differences between the professional approach and the self-help way and to observe their dialectical opposition. A meaningful synthesis can emerge only if we include saying no as well as saying yes. Therefore, we will conduct an ideal type comparison of the professional and the self-help modalities, based on various sources (Derber, Schwartz, and Magrass, 1990; Gouldner, 1960; and Brint, 1994). Some current examples of the integration of the professional and self-help modes are then presented, further details of which are documented in later chapters (the AA model in Chapter Three, the mental health consumer in Chapter Five, and the peer school-based model in Chapter Six).

Most of the illustrations are drawn from mutual support groups, rather than self-help writ large. However, it should be noted that professional involvement is also operative in relation to the various forms of self-help: for example, self-help books are written and marketed primarily by professionals, self-care techniques originate with professionals, and school-based peer groups are trained and supervised by professional counselors and similar personnel. And then there are the huge number of groups, generally called support groups, that are organized and led by professional social workers, psychologists, and health educators.

The final portion of this chapter considers some of the issues raised by the California findings and proposes training specifically directed at professionals to assist them in their new roles. Concomitantly, some warning signals are offered to self-helpers regarding potential dangers inherent in the new combinations.

Positive syntheses of the self-help and professional modes may take many forms and can add significantly to the resources needed to expand and revitalize human services—our major theme. After all, no matter how effective and valuable self-help groups may be, at best they touch only a tiny portion of the populations in need, be they chronic patients, widows, or victims of abuse.

Help Versus Practice

Professional practice is based on systematic knowledge and scientific methodology and is contextualized by the fact that the help provided is a commodity to be bought, sold, and marketed. Derber and colleagues (1990) refer to this as the privatization of knowledge.[1] This dimension affects every phase of professional practice, sometimes overtly, sometimes subtly. But it is always present—and often overlooked.

The help provided by mutual aid groups, by contrast, is given free of charge (no longer treating help as a commodity to be bought and sold is known as *decommodification*) and is generally based on less systematic knowledge and conscious use of methodology. Rather, it is based on experience or codified procedures (like AA's twelve steps). Furthermore, it is rooted in the experience of people who have had the problem and who have developed ways of giving each other help. Simple and self-evident as this concept may be, the implications are important for understanding the nature of self-help.

Because self-help does not bow to the constraints of the market, it can develop helping combinations and patterns in fresh and original ways, unencumbered by professional assumptions. So, for example, retarded twenty-year-olds can function as caregivers for small children, burned-out professionals can provide mutual support for each other, and offenders and their victims can meet and talk.

The help given is not subject to the constraints of time, place, or format. It can be a twenty-four-hour-a-day hot line, a buddy on call at any time, immediate concrete assistance as well as emotional help, a three-hour meeting, or a five-minute telephone call. It can take place in a basement, in an apartment, on a street corner, in a community center, in a church, in an office, on a boat, at a fair, in a schoolroom, in a hospital, or in a funeral parlor.

The potential integration or synthesis of self-help and professional intervention styles should not obscure the differences or the useful conflict between the two approaches. Not only do practitioners of each learn from one other, but they unlearn as well, for in many cases they are held back by "trained incapacities." Moreover, integration does not mean that one discipline becomes the other. So, for example, when we hear people say that psychotherapists should share totally with their patients, we reject this surrender of the professional role because we do not believe that therapy should be identical with a mutual aid group. Each side of the dialectical equation must maintain its identity in order for new syntheses to emerge.

Both the professional model and the self-help model clearly have their own strengths and weaknesses. From this perspective, the tension between the two can be a positive force, even a creative force, helping to construct a dialectic that, on the one hand, encourages self-helpers to perceive the subjectivity of their system more clearly and, on the other hand, allows professionals to break the icy shell of formalism and monetary orientation that may distance them from the consumers they work with.

The goal being advocated here is not to dilute or minimize professionalism but rather to maximize its effectiveness by integrating it with elements of self-help practice and self-help ideology, a blending that ultimately could benefit both practitioner and client alike.

The difference in the two approaches should not be ignored, nor can it be resolved easily. Both partners will have to tolerate the process.

Professionalism Versus Self-Help

What elements make up the professional-help model? In what fundamental ways does it differ from the self-help prototype?

Traditionally speaking, professionalism is characterized by the following features:

1. A stress on the importance of protecting the practitioner's knowledge and practice from outsiders and nonprofessionals, the noncredentialized, the unlicensed

2. A rigorous system of controls that governs who is qualified to enter the profession

3. A collegial rather than a client-oriented center of focus; by implication, this means that any philosophical, theoretical, or structural change that takes place in a professional discipline comes primarily from within the discipline itself and not from the people who are served by it (quacks, it is interesting to note, have been defined as people who please their patients but not their colleagues)

4. The power in any client-professional relationship resides with the professional, and the relationship must be based on an irreversible teacher-student, doctor-patient, well person–sick person, helper-helpee formula; the client is the member of this unequal partnership who needs to learn, heal, see things more clearly, and make appropriate changes for the better

5. An emphasis on objectivity as an aim—especially important for understanding the professional ethos in general

In brief, the attitude adopted by most professionals is one of emotional detachment and scientific impartiality.

Indeed, in most cases of applied human help, one cannot but suppose that the best way of approaching the matter is via a path that threads its way between the extremes of objectivity stripped of feeling and a sentimental subjectivity devoid of all discrimination.

The knowledge that empowers self-help is both subjective and experiential. It comes from the heart and the gut and from personal encounters with the problem at hand. (One group member brought this point home at a self-help meeting by quoting Zsa Zsa Gabor's observation that "you never really know a man until you divorce him.")

Professional knowledge, by contrast, is based not on personal experience but on research, empirical observations, and the analysis of other people's personal experience, which is in turn gained by experiment, a system of controls, and controlled observation.

Clearly, such an approach has great potential value in the human helping process, both in terms of gaining clarity about certain behaviors and in reducing the negative effects of bias.

The fact is that many professionals maintain an interest in promoting their knowledge, theories, training, reputation, and credentials. Because professionals sell this knowledge in the marketplace rather than dispense it on a free and egalitarian basis as in a self-help group, the temptations are strong to exaggerate its effectiveness, monopolize its best features, prolong its application to clients, manufacture an arcane jargon to make it impenetrable to the uninitiated, and construct duchies of power around it to wall this knowledge off from outside criticism and change. Such behavior compromises objectivity.

A perfect example of compromised professionalism is the forty-five-minute session schedule presently used by psychotherapists and psychiatrists. In the early days, therapists spent a full hour with their clients. Such work was extremely intense, however, and practitioners found that they needed a five-minute break between visits. The fifty-five-minute hour was born.

As more time passed, professionals determined that what they really needed was a ten-minute break, and soon that expanded to a fifteen-minute break.

They deserved it. Therapy is grueling work. The trouble was, one day a clever therapist came along and started scheduling patients for back-to-back forty-five-minute visits with no break in between, thus making a mockery of the original reason for having a rest period and thereby decreasing the quality of service delivered to clients in direct ratio to increasing monetary gain. Before long, other therapists were imitating the same model.

This ploy stands as a metaphor not only of professional abuse of power but also of the contrast between the professional ethic and the ethic of self-help in general. Table 2.1 spells this contrast out in detail. There is no doubt that both disciplines contain a vivid and healing message and that each offers important features that the other lacks.

From the self-help perspective, human services should be centered on the client, or consumer; and in the end, it is the client who

Table 2.1. Comparison of Professional and Mutual Aid Models.

Professional Model	Mutual Aid Model
1. Doctor knows best. Don't try to treat yourself; you'll only make things worse. Objective outside expertise is required to diagnose and remedy all social, medical, or psychological problems. Self-treatment is ineffective and possibly dangerous.	1. Self-help is also self-treatment. Individuals know best what they need, and they recognize this help when they see it. Real help ultimately comes from within rather than without—all the outside input can do is stimulate the inner self-healing mechanism.
2. Emphasis on training, credentials, and education. Belief that if you have not undergone this training, you are not qualified to play the role of teacher. Implication that the professional has the knowledge and depth to understand and treat human problems. Helping knowledge reposes exclusively in official organizations, agencies, and institutions: universities, teaching centers, hospitals, clinics, psychiatric and health care facilities, rehabilitation centers, and human service organizations.	2. No special qualifications for admission. Nonselective membership policies. Everyone is welcome to participate (though there are no guarantees that they will be listened to). All members have the right to contribute, regardless of education or background. (Conversely, no member is obliged to do what another says if the advice seems skewed or incorrect.) Qualifications for expertise are based on experience, role modeling, and usefulness of help offered.

Table 2.1. *Continued*

Professional Model	Mutual Aid Model
3. The professional is the source of power in the relationship; all dealings between patient and professional flow along hierarchical lines.	3. Power is distributed throughout the group in an even and egalitarian way. Leadership positions are interchangeable or rotating. Power flows in a horizontal rather than a vertical or hierarchical way. Everyone owns a share in the collective power base. No charismatic leadership.
4. Help is sold to patients as a commodity. Fees are received for a professional's time and expertise, and help stops if this payment is not forthcoming.	4. Service is given as a voluntary act or as a means of attaining self-improvement. No fee or admission is charged. Money may be regarded as a potentially corrupting influence within the group structure.
5. Help provision is viewed exclusively as a job or profession.	5. Help provision is looked on as a community service, a good deed, an energy-releasing activity, and an ongoing, twenty-four-hour-a-day human responsibility.
6. Emphasis is on an underlying approach. The professional attempts to be objective. Treatment is based on research, empirical observation, and an established set of theories.	6. Emphasis is on the subjective and spontaneous response: common sense, intuition, gut reaction, folk wisdom, and direct experience. Focus is on dealing with present-time, day-to-day issues.
7. The professional is nonjudgmental and nonconfrontational.	7. Members may criticize one another or enter into overtly confrontational behavior. Interpersonal conflict is allowed, if not encouraged. Advice and counsel are freely given, sometimes even when unsolicited.

Table 2.1. *Continued*

Professional Model	Mutual Aid Model
8. Professionals act neither as peers nor as role models for their patients. Socializing or friendship in the help-giving relationship session is discouraged. In times of crisis, telephone help or extra (paid) sessions are offered. Professionals remain non-self-revealing. Meetings are held in formal settings such as hospitals, offices, clinics, and health care suites according to a definite schedule.	8. Members are encouraged to socialize and continue providing help for one another outside meetings. Members remain in contact and are available in time of crisis. Self-revelation, honesty, and sharing among participants is looked on as commendatory. Meetings are held in any convenient public or private location such as a school, home, or community center.

must produce his or her own health and well-being. (It has in fact been estimated that 85 percent of all health care in this country is self-care; Levin, Katz, and Holtz, 1976).

This is not to deny that the self-help movement possesses its own set of perplexities, inconsistencies, and flaws. These often derive from a lack of the very qualities—objectivity, systematic knowledge, trained leadership—that give the professional approach its helping power.

For example, visitors to mutual aid meetings are often bothered by the overly subjective and sometimes embarrassingly personal tone of the exchanges that take place. A variety of advice and opinions are traded, some relevant, some marginal, some quite bizarre. Indeed, the very tolerance that welcomes all members and allows each to have a say can at times end up encouraging meandering monologues, attention hogging, and irrelevant bickering. Meanwhile, the accountability level for such antics remains disturbingly low.

Because admission is free and nonselective at self-help groups, visits from individuals with self-serving or even hostile agendas are not unheard of.

And because many self-help organizations avoid espousing a systematic doctrine, meetings sometimes have an unfocused and even chaotic air. Intuition, feelings, gut responses—all highly prized by self-helpers—at times exceed their limits, turning into maudlin overindulgence and excessive emotionalism. There is often no one in attendance with the skill to steer the group away from trivial or disruptive matters and toward the issues that count. What is more, if the leadership of the group is undefined or revolving, certain members may maneuver themselves into dominant positions by sheer force of personality and podium grabbing until they co-opt a majority of the power without assuming any of the accountability.

In short, the very qualities that foster self-help empowerment—democratic spirit, sharing, free and open admission, emotional support, and reciprocal leadership—can turn out to be the self-help movement's most serious detriments.

The self-help movement offers new lessons, new services, new models, new techniques, and a high degree of original thinking that we believe professionals in all disciplines would be well advised to heed.

At the same time, the professional model has a number of impressive strengths of its own that must not be sacrificed. Expert training, skilled leadership abilities, systematic knowledge, commitment to service, and a broad intellectual perspective are all important features that the self-help world often ignores or even belittles but may ultimately prove crucial to self-transformation.

Courting Common Ground

Although the differences between the professional and self-help ideologies are substantial, they are not wholly incompatible. In fact, the two camps share common ground. This point is often missed and is worth examining.

First, of course, is the fact that both methodologies exist to help, serve, and heal people. This is a powerful shared ambition that of itself forges a robust bond between the two disciplines.

Second, both self-help and professionals may share a common enemy: bureaucracy. For both disciplines, independence from the restrictions, officialism, and red tape that have brought so many worthy causes to their knees is a common goal, one for which alliances are often formed.

Finally, although the methods practiced by professionals and self-help groups differ in form and philosophy, they are by no means mutually exclusive and sometimes even supplement one another.

Certainly the relationship of AAers with professional services is a case in point. Here a number of for-pay rehabilitation centers staffed by doctors and other professionals have incorporated twelve-step philosophy into their treatment strategy, hired sober alcoholics as instructors, and urged patients to participate in AA meetings as part of their treatment. The result is a seamless combination of the best elements of professionalism and the methods of self-help. Many similar instances exist, several of which we will detail in Chapter Three.

These and other common linkages, moreover, have made their presence known in a number of crossover and handshake influences.

Through the years, for example, professionals have related to the self-help movement by sending clients to self-help groups or by recruiting clients from these groups for their own practice. Many professionals are increasingly willing to accept and encourage mutual self-help organizations, even though these organizations appear to represent competition. Likewise, more and more professionals provide self-help organizations with research materials and technical data. They furnish short-term leadership training and serve in an advisory or consultative role. At times they lend advice on the intricacies of private and government fundraising, help design and evaluate studies, and contribute to self-help books and journals. Especially in the medical and mental health fields, professionals who perceive that a certain area of care is failing to receive the attention it deserves may set up a support group on their own.

Though many professionals seem to view the self-help movement as the stepchild of the helping services, there is at the same time definite movement between the two worlds toward what former Surgeon General C. Everett Koop referred to as "a growing partnership" (U.S. Department of Health and Human Services, 1987, p. 4). This partnership consists of such elements as professionals designing and evaluating studies of self-help groups, delivering periodic lectures at self-help meetings, periodically observing and consulting at meetings, writing self-help magazine articles and books, and providing intragroup training. All these activities give back as much as they take, broadening professional experience and adding to the participants' knowledge base. Recent studies have shown not only generally positive attitudes toward professionals and agencies by self-help group members but also that members increase their use of professional services after experience in self-help groups. These effects have occurred despite the fact that some groups were created after disappointing experiences with professionals or out of a conviction that needs were not being adequately met (Katz, 1987, p. 33).

In the ideal model, professionals can serve as external aids in relation to the internal resources, needs, strengths, and activities of the group. Professionals accomplish this feat, first, by playing the role of facilitator and trainer and, second, by providing the group with external resources such as knowledge, research materials, funding sources, organization, networks, and political contacts.

In the health care arena, for example, a vast industry of self-help books, teaching cassettes, telephone help lines, interactive computer software, on-line programs, consumer organizations, annual conferences, advocacy movements, home care agencies, alternative self-treatment medical techniques (such as acupressure, massage, reflexology, and herbalism), and do-it-yourself medical apparatus (such as self-applied pregnancy tests, urine sticks to estimate sugar levels, colon-screening tests, home orthopedic devices, and home blood pressure–measuring instruments) have sprung up as a result of the collaboration between self-help and health care professionals. These products, services, and agencies can be viewed as part of the health system's self-care armamentarium, designed to be used in concert with self-help philosophy.

Cooperation Illustrated

Even more central to our purpose is the question of efficacy. What real-world examples of cooperation between professionals and mutual aid groups can serve as models for us to study, learn from, and perhaps emulate? Let us look at some cases that show how the two methodologies can be brought together to create a synergistic force that makes the best use of both systems.

Addiction, Acupuncture, and Self-Help

An innovative anti–substance abuse program is currently functioning at Lincoln Hospital, in a black and Latino area of the South Bronx in New York City. Since 1974, the hospital's acupuncture staff, led by Dr. Michael Smith, has been using acupuncture therapy to treat severe addictions to alcohol, heroin, Valium, PCP, and cocaine.

Hard-core addicts are often surprised to discover that daily acupuncture treatments relieve withdrawal symptoms without producing unpleasant side effects or addiction to chemical substitutes. The Lincoln Hospital acupuncture project has been so successful, in fact, that it has inspired similar programs in thirty cities.

What makes this program unique, beside the fact that it uses an alternative medical technique in a conventional medical setting, is that as part of the program, the participants are urged to join a local branch of Narcotics Anonymous or Alcoholics Anonymous. Meetings of both organizations are even held for patients in the hospital itself.

One NA group consists of young mothers who attend the clinic every day with their infants and children. A three-month follow-up of women with "crack babies" who were referred to the Lincoln Hospital Clinic by the New York Department of Social Services determined that 55 percent of these women were attending NA meetings on a regular basis. According to Smith, "Referral to these twelve-step programs is an important part of our counseling and overall treatment program. Our focus on the priority of drug-free behavior fits well with their approach. NA and AA ask their members to hold on to sobriety one day at a time and to rely on the network of support of fellow members" (personal correspondence with author, September 10, 1994).

Consumer-Led Mental Health Services

The Community Support Program (CSP), a project of the National Institute of Mental Health, has sponsored and funded an extremely interesting approach to mental self-help over the past several decades. The concept is a simple one: ex–mental patients (former *consumers* of mental health services) are "recycled" and employed as aides and administrators (as *producers* of mental health services) to provide services for current psychiatric patients (see Chapter Five).

In Philadelphia, Project SHARE, a consumer-intensive case management project, employs former mental health patients as paid case managers. All participants complete a full course of study at Temple University and are specially trained. Employees in this program carry beepers and are on call twenty-four hours a day. Clinical supervision is provided by a director, an experienced mental health clinician, and a former consumer of mental health services. The program emphasizes self-governance and a reduction of distinctions between caregivers and clients.

A similar project, Denver's Consumer Case Management Program, was launched in 1987 with funds from the Federal Job Training Partnership Act and the Colorado Department of Mental Health. This far-seeing venture employs twenty-five former mental health patients specially trained at the Community College of Denver to serve as case workers for four hundred clients of Denver's

Mental Health Corporation. Emphasis in the program is on offering clients role models, interpersonal contact, and help in coping with the exigencies of everyday living.

Studies confirm that such programs are of substantial benefit in increasing work productivity and in lengthening the time that patients are able to live on their own without requiring hospitalization (*Harvard*, 1992).

Professional Group Leadership Training

Laurieann Chutis, a mental health professional who works at Ravenswood Hospital Community Mental Health Center in Chicago, perceived a need at her clinic for increased patient participation. So she developed a self-help group leadership training methodology suitable for a spectrum of populations, including widowed people, incest survivors, adult children of alcoholics, compulsive eaters, and victims of rape.

Her training program follows a seven-step plan that, in a nutshell, involves sharing information and resources, group relaxation exercises, confidentiality, discussion of approved topics (always of a personal nature and relevance to the group), and roundtable sharing of feelings and ideas. Her work is typical of that of other professionals in clinical settings who have become aware of unfulfilled needs among their institutions' patient populations and have addressed them using the self-help model as guide.

Parents Anonymous

An extremely interesting amalgam of self-help and professionalism in the crisis intervention area is Parents Anonymous (PA), a non-twelve-step self-help group that caters to parents who abuse, neglect, or otherwise mistreat their children.

Founded in 1970 by Leonard Leiber, a professional social worker, and a patient of his named Jolly, Parents Anonymous today has twelve hundred groups across the country, all of which are peer-led but include professional sponsors. Members of PA are taught to relate to and discipline their children in nonviolent ways. They are guided to express their feelings in positive terms and to make life changes that improve family relationships. As in the self-help model, attendance at meetings is free.

Members also work with the professional sponsors, and group-run information hot lines refer inquiring persons to professional therapists or agencies. PA likewise sponsors professionally facilitated self-help groups for abused children.

School-Centered Peer Groups

One of the most successful interventions in schools today centers around a one-on-one system of peer help whereby students counsel, tutor, or advise other youngsters their own age (or younger) on such topics as sex, drug abuse, and schoolwork. This interaction involves the application of basic self-help principles—the use of internal resources—without the term *self-help* being applied.

Peer programs are facilitated by professional teachers or counselors who train peer counselors and oversee their activities. (The peer approach is discussed at length in Chapter Six.)

SHARE (Self-Help for Women with Breast Cancer)

In many cases, professional involvement with a self-help group may be time-limited. This involvement is often at the beginning, when a group is starting and may require the skills of a professional to get it past the hurdles.

In such cases, the professional helps organize the group, sets up a schedule, establishes an agenda and a modus operandi, oversees meetings for a period of time, and then, when satisfied that the group has become self-sufficient, recedes into the background, becoming a consultant or a member of the board.

A case in point is SHARE, a self-help group founded by Dr. Eugene Thyssen to help women cope with the psychological aftershock of mastectomy. Realizing that he alone was not able to provide the emotional care and support necessary for postmastectomy patients—and understanding that such help comes best through the mutual sharing of experiences within a group dynamic—Thyssen helped found SHARE, recruited members, oversaw its early days, and then relinquished control and allowed the group to run itself.

Doctor-Sponsored Medical Self-Care

Although many physicians continue to resist patient-administered care and certain powerful medical associations seem determined to keep patients as far removed from their own medical treatment as possible—even in instances where self-care is practicable, advisable, and cost-effective—a grassroots alliance among physicians and disease-oriented self-help groups is growing. Indeed, a small but powerful movement is emerging from within the medical community itself, sponsored by doctors, nurses, and health care workers, all of whom advocate increased patient participation and education.

Patient awareness groups, led by physicians and paramedics around the country, currently teach participants the fundamentals of medical self-care for minor problems and complaints. This increased knowledge on the part of patients in turn frees doctors to help patients suffering from more serious ailments. Thus, as in any good self-help ecosystem, consumers become producers, and resources are allocated more efficiently throughout the system.

Literature on the subject of medical self-care is likewise appearing with increasing frequency, even in the most conservative medical journals, and industries of all kinds produce more than a billion dollars' worth of home-care medical self-tests and equipment each year. Popular magazines such as *Medical Self-Care* regularly feature articles on self-care written by nurses and physicians amenable to the concept of patient empowerment. *Medical Self-Care* publishes a comprehensive state-by-state directory of physicians, nurses, and therapists who encourage self-care and who participate in self-health maintenance programs and educational groups. Similar efforts combining patient advocacy and medical professionalism are taking place throughout the country.

Family Intervention

Donald H. was drinking heavily, teetering on the edge of alcoholic self-destruction. He had been fired several times for being drunk on the job, one of his children had left home to escape him, and his marriage was deeply troubled. Encouraged by his wife to visit a therapist, it became apparent after several months of treatment that Donald was indeed attempting to drink his problems away and was desperately in need of rehabilitation.

When confronted by his therapist, however, Donald balked. In his mind there was no problem at all, period. Things were fine as they were, just fine, and needed no fixing. Nor did the entreaties of his friends and family help him see things differently. Donald was in denial.

Realizing that Donald's fate hung in the balance and that he was unable to recognize the seriousness of his situation, the therapist did three things. First, she contacted a rehabilitation center she had worked with in the past. Second, she contacted a friend at AA. Third, she arranged a surprise family intervention.

One rainy Sunday, lured to a hotel room by an uncle who had invited him to dinner, Donald entered to find his entire family waiting for him—mother, father, wife, her daughter, and their two children, plus assorted uncles, aunts, and cousins. Each in turn read Donald a written statement spelling out the problems that his drinking had caused them and beseeching him to quit.

Moved and shaken by this experience, Donald agreed on the spot to seek help. Thanks to the preliminary work already done by the therapist, the rehabilitation center had a bed waiting for him. During rehabilitation and after, Donald attended AA meetings and participated in AA activities.

In this case, the therapist succeeded in skillfully combining several powerful interventions into one, taking advantage of therapy, group help, professional rehabilitation facilities, and Alcoholics Anonymous. The result was that today Donald is sober, working, still married, and an active member of his local AA group.

Implications

What are the implications of the increased involvement of professionals in mutual self-help groups? Goodman and Jacobs report that professionals serve in thirteen different capacities. In 14 percent of groups, a professional serves as sole leader; in another 35 percent, they are joint leaders, along with—or alternating with—a member of the group (Goodman and Jacobs, 1994, p. 496).

Although the most common form of professional involvement is referring new members to the self-help groups, in 38 percent of the sample, professionals participated as regular members. In addition, professionals are frequently brought in as speakers and function as consultants or advisers on problems such as group process. Professionals also help line up meeting places and other resources for the group and function as observers and "evaluators."

Goodman and Jacobs observe that most of these activities are welcomed by the self-help groups and that they desire even more involvement by professionals as speakers, teachers, students, and coleaders. The self-help respondents were least interested in having professionals serve as solo leaders or coordinator-organizers. However, the data suggest that in 37 percent of the groups, professionals intervened less than two hours a month. Twenty percent of the groups reported professional involvement of ten hours a month, and only 10 percent reported more. What are the implications?

1. On the positive side, we can anticipate the blending of two avenues to help and a possible creative synthesis, particularly

if the leadership of these groups genuinely remains in the hands of the group members and the group members are themselves individuals who share the central problem or concern of the group. There is the possibility, of course, that professionals participating in self-help groups may simply be functioning in their professional roles, thus diluting the self-help groups. The fact that a good number of these professionals are employed by social agencies also tends to work against the decommodification principle.

2. There is the danger that the professional orientation or style may increasingly dominate the groups. Because not much training in most graduate programs (or in the agencies) is directed at understanding and working with self-help groups, we might anticipate some combination of strife and confusion, along with potential efforts at professional control and co-optation. Depending on the ethos strength of the groups, they might become miniature group therapy sessions.

3. It will be important to know the stance of the professionals with regard to the self-help groups and their roles in the groups. Do they have a high regard for self-help and its ethos? Do they see themselves as facilitators, not major players? Do they perceive the need for training? Is an important motive the obtaining of clients for themselves or their agencies? Do they view professional knowledge as that of a higher order to be protected and perhaps mystified, or do they wish to share it with their new partners? How much tension and conflict are the professionals prepared to tolerate? How able are they to learn from the self-helpers' experiential knowledge base? And finally, do they see themselves as temporary part-time aides or as long-term full participants?

As we have seen, there are various models of professional self-help interaction, ranging from peer groups in schools—in which training and management are entirely in the hands of profession-als—to groups of mental health consumers running programs.

All of this leads to the issue of training on the job and in grad-uate schools. Training is rarely independent of stance. If the stance is one of respect for the independence, self-determination, and experiential knowledge base of the self-help group, the training of the professional will be very different than if the focus is on influ-encing the group. In the former instance, the following model may be relevant.

Training Professionals

The following are suggestions for training professionals to work with self-help groups (Dory and Riessman, 1982; see also Cardinal and Farquharson, 1991):

- Have professionals attend open meetings of existing self-help groups.

- Simulate self-help groups in the training process.

- Have some sessions in the training process include members of self-help groups, films of self-help groups, or presentations by members of self-help groups.

- Have discussions of the "self-help way" in contrast to the professional way and away from the need to control the group.

- Present case histories of professionals working with self-help groups, with particular emphasis on various critical decision points, such as entry, developing a contract, or dealing with a group that is stuck.

- Help the professional accept that there is a natural, useful tension between self-help groups and profes-sionals.

• Help the professional learn to spot leadership and encourage it.

• Conduct most of the training in an experiential fashion with a minimum of didactic presentation.

• Help the professional assess the organizational setting in which he or she works and the issues involved in introducing self-help groups in the particular setting—how to overcome resistance and develop strategy.

• Review the many ways in which professionals have related to self-help groups and provide various examples (Parents Anonymous, peer-counseling groups, SHARE, widows' groups, Families of the Mentally Ill, Compassionate Friends, Mended Hearts, the Fortune Society).

• Encourage the professional to join a self-help group and to reflect on this participation, as well as participation in other self-help groups of which he or she was a member, or to form a group to deal with his or her own issues of burnout.

Conclusion

There is no question that this new mix of professionals and self-helpers has great potential for expanding the resources for human services, but there are dangers for the self-help movement that will require considerable alertness to mitigate or overcome. These dangers arise from two sources: (1) the privatization-of-knowledge perspective, characteristic of professionals, as it plays itself out in relation to the free giving of help, characteristic of the self-help mode, and (2) the clash of the experiential orientation of self-help with the professional orientation attuned to formal knowledge. The latter may not be provided to self-helpers (this relates, of course, to the first point). As Derber and colleagues note, the self-help movement is a critical consumer constituency implicitly calling for the democratization of knowledge. Thus professional–self-help integration may well be one of the battlegrounds for this larger issue, and the stance and training of professionals working with self-help groups are of critical importance.

Goodwill alone will probably not suffice because of professionals' historical tendency to control the dispensing of help or service in relation to their own monetary and status interests. Knowledge is privatized for this reason, and that must be understood by both the self-helpers and well-meaning professionals themselves. To be truly well-meaning, the professionals will have to be open to the democratization of knowledge and to experience-based knowledge; it can be a natural boon to their own development. Certainly, it seems to us that for a long transitional period, the engagement of professionals in self-help activities should be limited in time and intensity, perhaps to consulting and facilitating rather than leading.

The Special Significance of the Alcoholics Anonymous Model

The special significance of AA is based on two factors: (1) its impact on mainstream human services—no other self-help system has had this kind of influence—and its comprehensiveness, including the theoretical structure for interpreting the phenomenon of alcoholism and its intervention rationale, broad infrastructure of help, and remarkable organizational model. It is for these reasons that we give special attention to the AA system, which may have broad implications for the self-help movement as a whole.

The Beginning

May 1935. Mayflower Hotel, Akron, Ohio. A pale, tired-looking man named Bill Wilson is pacing the lobby, frantic for a drink. At the end of the corridor, the hotel bar rings with laughter and the sound of ice in a glass. Bill keeps eyeing it. An important stock deal has just fallen through, and the only way he knows of drowning his sorrows is the bottle.

The trouble is, he's been sober now for six months, and he's well aware that one slip, one sip, will put him face to face with the d.t.'s. He paces the lobby remembering the dry-out tanks in his hometown sanitarium, the moralizing pep talks from the nurses and the doctors and just about everyone. He remembers his trips home from the hospital feeling appropriately repentant and eager to turn over a new leaf. After that, straight for a day, for a week, for a month, then back to the tanks for yet another round of treatment, world without end.

Now here he is, far from home and late at night, sober in a hotel lobby, with every cell in his body screaming for alcohol. The lights of the bar call him over for a friendly nightcap. Just one. He starts to walk in their direction. Just as he reaches the doorway, a billboard displaying a list of churches and ministers in the Akron area catches his eye. With a superhuman effort, he stops in his tracks, jots down the first name he sees on the board, goes to a phone booth, and calls a perfect stranger for help.

On this night, with this call, the first self-help group was born.

The rest of the story is a familiar one. A certain Reverend Tunks directs his late-night caller to a physician named Bob Smith. The two men meet, talk, and quickly discover that they share the same penchant for alcoholic self-destruction. Perhaps if they get together on a regular basis to trade experiences, to serve as mutual watchdog and nursemaid, to play adviser and advisee to each other in turn; perhaps if they follow their own gut feelings rather than the for-hire advice of purported experts; perhaps if they help each other—just perhaps—they can lick this monster together.

And so they agreed.

That was it; that was all. Yet this arrangement would set off a chain of events leading to the eventual foundation of Alcoholics Anonymous. What Bill Wilson discovered was that perhaps alcoholics needed a drunk rather than a drink.

AA itself arose out of the recognition that organized medicine had failed dismally in its understanding and treatment of alcoholism. Given the sea change in popular awareness of the problem and the enormous strides in treatment, it may be difficult today to appreciate what it was like for alcoholics in the 1930s and 1940s when AA was still in its early organizing stages. Most hospitals would not admit alcoholics; treatment was to be found only at a handful of large hospitals, whose drying-out facilities were so expensive that few people could afford them.

From the beginning, Bill Wilson and the other AA pioneers realized the importance of removing the stigma from alcoholism. People should view alcoholism as a disease, he reasoned, like any other, and not as a fatal flaw of character or a symptom of moral weakness. This disease concept was to prove extremely useful in treatment, lifting a large burden of guilt from both patient and family and allowing the work of recovery to focus on the self-help mutual aid group.

Whatever one ultimately thinks of Alcoholics Anonymous, it is obvious that the twelve-step approach developed by its founders (see Exhibit 3.1) has worked its way into our national consciousness on many levels. Common words and phrases (*anonymity, sponsor, Higher Power, easy does it, one day at a time*) given special connotative meanings by AA are now part of the language. AA meetings are a regular occurrence at churches, schools, town halls, and community centers. References to its activities are common in all branches of the media. A number of its techniques have been adopted by professional therapists and by twelve-step recovery centers.

Moreover, of the hundred or more types of twelve-step programs currently playing host to over two million Americans from Bangor to Spokane, almost every one counts itself a spiritual child of AA. These programs cater to a great variety of addictions—Gamblers Anonymous, Debtors Anonymous, Overeaters Anonymous—and all have taken AA as their living model.

The First Meeting

What happens to an alcoholic on his first encounter with A.A. is that he realizes he has been invited to share in the experience of recovery, . . . and that he has been invited to share as an equal and not as a medicant. . . . And he is made to feel that he is, in fact, *entitled* to all this—indeed, he has already earned it—simply because he is an alcoholic. . . .

Much more important than *what* . . . [was] said . . . [is] . . . *who* was saying it. Long before the average alcoholic

Exhibit 3.1. The Twelve Suggested Steps of Alcoholics Anonymous.

1. We admitted we were powerless over alcohol—that our lives had become unmanageable.

2. Came to believe that a Power greater than ourselves could restore us to sanity.

3. Made a decision to turn our will and our lives over to the care of God as we understood Him.

4. Made a searching and fearless moral inventory of ourselves.

5. Admitted to God, to ourselves, and to another human being the exact nature of our wrongs.

6. Were entirely ready to have God remove all these defects of character.

7. Humbly asked Him to remove our shortcomings.

8. Made a list of all persons we had harmed and became willing to make amends to them all.

9. Made direct amends to such people whenever possible, except when to do so would injure them or others.

10. Continued to take personal inventory and, when we were wrong, promptly admitted it.

11. Sought through prayer and meditation to improve our conscious contact with God, as we understood Him, praying only for knowledge of His will for us and the power to carry that out.

12. Having had a spiritual awakening as a result of these steps, we tried to carry this message to alcoholics and to practice these principles in all our affairs.

walks through the doors of his first A.A. meeting, he has
sought help from others or help has been offered to him,
in some instances even forced upon him. But these
helpers are always superior beings: . . . parents, physicians, employers, priests, ministers, rabbis, swamis,
judges, policemen, even bartenders. The moral culpabil-
ity of the alcoholic and the moral superiority of the
helper, even though unstated, are always clearly understood. . . . For the first time, 33 years ago an alcoholic
suddenly heard a different drummer. Instead of the constant and menacing rat-a-tat-tat of "This is what you
should do," he heard an instantly recognizable voice saying, "This is what I did" (*Member's Eye View*, p. 10).

From Abstinence to Sobriety

The only official requirement for joining Alcoholics Anonymous is
the desire to stop drinking. Yet once signed on and committed,
members soon discover that AA's goals are a good deal more ambi-
tious than its brochures may lead them to believe and that its aim
is nothing less than the psychic refurbishment of the entire individual.

Its goal is sobriety, to be obtained through the twelve steps that
aim to transform the person. These steps include "making a searching and fearless moral inventory," "making amends to people one
has harmed," and an overall spiritual awakening that might be
termed a reduction of narcissistic ego together with a concern and
caring for others—in other words, becoming a better total person.

Abstinence puts a tremendous strain on the individual, but
sobriety, stemming as it does from a larger transformation of the
individual, allows the alcoholic to remain sober as a life pattern,
one that is deemed necessary because the alcoholism is viewed as
an underlying disease that does not permit the intake of alcohol,
even in moderation.

The full significance of this transformation is reflected in "The Promises" from *Alcoholics Anonymous*:

> We are going to know a new freedom and a new happiness. We will not neglect the past nor [do we] wish to shut the door on it. We will comprehend the word serenity and will know peace. No matter how far down the scale we have gone, we will see how our experience can benefit others. The feeling of uselessness and self-pity will disappear. We will lose interest in selfish things and gain interest in our fellows. Self-seeking will slip away. Our whole attitude on life will leave us. We will intuitively know how to handle situations which used to baffle us (Wilson, 1939, p. 77).

Any evaluation that compares AA with other interventions in terms of abstinence alone misses the mark because it is these other dimensions that account for the holding power of AA, the intense commitment to it. This commitment is not simply based on the participants' remaining sober but rather on what AA calls spirituality, which, one writer explains, "is not synonymous with religion. . . . Spirituality is simply an awareness that you are not the center of the universe; it is an intuitive sense of a vital principle or animating force. It . . . [is] the apprehension that there is something more" (Mundis, 1990, pp. 287–289). Another observes that spirituality is "a powerful agent of centering, of peace and serenity. . . . Developing it is basically a process of letting go of self-will. That doesn't mean abdicating responsibility. . . . It means recognizing and admitting that you don't have all the answers, . . . that you are not God. . . . It is a willingness to trust what is best in yourself" (Kurtz and Ketcham, 1992, p. 287).

The spiritual dimension is one of the most perplexing aspects of AA to outsiders. Many researchers are surprised to find enthusiastic membership in self-help groups with relatively small improvements in the physical condition of the illness. What they fail to understand is that the self-help group itself provides a kind of spiritual community for its members.

This carefully worked out spiritual program at AA makes clear the fundamental difference between ordinary *abstinence*, as championed by non-twelve-step programs, and *sobriety*, which for AA members bears a highly defined meaning and connotation.

Ordinary abstinence, in this sense, is enforced self-denial, a voluntary and painful act of renunciation that conjures up images of herculean personal efforts made against the very forces of nature itself. By contrast, sobriety, as understood by AA members, is not an isolated act of denial or the result of superhuman will. It is a natural and inevitable *end product* of a greater process of spiritual inner transformation that takes place as a matter of course, by following AA's mandates. In AA, a person who has successfully followed the program is assumed to be—there is no better word for it—reborn.

What is the price of this redemption? Members are exhorted never to drink again. Alcoholism is regarded as a physiological disease caused and exacerbated by alcohol. Medically speaking, members must avoid its use for the rest of their lives, even in moderation, or pay the price. Even one drink is too many. Indeed, for the committed AA member, any drinking at all is a doctrinal impossibility.

All of these matters considered, we can now see that critics who attempt to take AA to task for its idiosyncratic methods and who spend time penning theses on why AA is less effective than other non-twelve-step interventions are missing the point.

The point is simply this: that the features of Alcoholics Anonymous that its critics attack so vociferously and that set it off from conventional modalities—the seven-day-a-week meeting schedules, a Sunday-go-to-meeting atmosphere, the demands for a lifetime commitment, the clannish closeness of members—are precisely the features that attract people so strongly and keep them so committed.

This commitment is not based solely on the attainment of sobriety (indeed, some AA members drink on a regular basis for years and still attend meetings). It is based, rather, on a spectrum of social and emotional benefits that members are lacking in other areas of their lives.

This bias explains why surprised researchers find some AA members (and some members of many other twelve-step groups) so deeply committed, even when there is little indication that their illness or addiction is improving. What these researchers fail to understand is that the group itself provides a sense of spiritual fellowship and support for its members that may be of equal or even greater importance to them than recovering from addiction.

The Tools of the Program

In addition to its spiritual component, the attraction of AA is based on its operational and organizational tools.

Good examples are the first two steps in the twelve-step tradition: the admission of powerlessness (over the urge to drink) and the belief that a Higher Power can help one recover from addiction.

The first step is empowering ("powerless empowerment") as it encourages individuals to accept their limits, stop blaming themselves for the things that cannot be helped or changed, and recognize that willpower alone is too small a slingshot to kill the Goliath of alcoholism. The second step promises that recovery is possible and that members will discover the path for themselves if they abide by the program.

These two steps are characteristic of the way AA transforms idealism into practical utensils of the self-help trade.

Witness other examples, too, such as the round-the-clock meetings, the daily readings, the ongoing group activities, the constant repetition of slogans ("Let Go—Let God," "Keep It Simple, Sweetheart," "Awareness, Acceptance, Action"), the assumption of new life responsibilities, the helping of other people, the preoccupation with acclimatizing oneself to a new way of thinking—these and other typical AA supports have a powerful stabilizing influence on people whose lives were once in ruins. When experienced in toto, they serve as a powerful builder of group solidarity, providing members with a structured way of life that in itself has a healing quality. Many addiction treatment programs that have borrowed from AA recognize the deep appeal of AA's tightly organized regimen.

Still another ingenious AA tool is the group itself, with its offerings of emotional support, collective wisdom, and a safety net for those who fall from the high wire of sobriety. Its power structure runs counter to the top-down hierarchy so prevalent in our society, providing members with a true grassroots democracy in which all citizens are equally listened to and equally anonymous—first names only is the rule—and each local group remains autonomous.

In the inner circle at these meetings, participants are encouraged to give help and accept it in equal measure. The unequal patient-physician relationship is exchanged for a more egalitarian one, a "peer-group democracy," if you will. Rather than be ruled over by disinterested professionals, the group roundtable consists of persons who have served their apprenticeship in addiction and who now draw on life experiences to guide others. ("The spiritual foundation of all our traditions ever reminds us to place principles before personalities.")

AA's organizational model is opposed to the bureaucratic hierarchies of most organizations. AA's structure is essentially democratic, with power diffused throughout the group. Leaders are viewed as trusted servants who do not govern and who, like everybody else, follow a code of anonymity. There is no charge for participation and no outlet for entrepreneurship or political self-aggrandizement. Above all, AA offers a system that manages to be both accessible and confidential.

Loyal chapters insist on maintaining an amateur status; according to the Twelve Traditions (see Exhibit 3.2), all groups are obliged by fellowship principles to "remain forever nonprofessional." Most refreshingly, in this age of megahype and galloping self-promotion, AA self-effacingly maintains a policy of "attraction rather than pro-

Exhibit 3.2. The Twelve Traditions of Alcoholics Anonymous.

1. Our common welfare should come first; personal recovery depends upon AA unity.

2. For our group purpose there is but one ultimate authority—a loving God as He may express Himself in our group conscience. Our leaders are but trusted servants; they do not govern.

3. The only requirement for AA membership is a desire to stop drinking.

4. Each group should be autonomous except in matters affecting other groups or AA as a whole.

5. Each group has but one primary purpose—to carry its message to the alcoholic who still suffers.

6. An AA group ought never to endorse, finance, or lend the AA name to any related facility or outside enterprise, lest problems of money, property, and prestige divert us from our primary purpose.

7. Every AA group ought to be fully self-supporting, declining outside contributions.

8. Alcoholics Anonymous should remain forever nonprofessional, but our service centers may employ special workers.

9. AA, as such, ought never to be organized; but we may create service boards or committees directly responsible to those they serve.

10. Alcoholics Anonymous has no opinion on outside issues; hence the AA name ought never to be drawn into public controversy.

11. Our public relations policy is based on attraction rather than promotion; we need always maintain personal anonymity at the level of press, radio, and films.

12. Anonymity is the spiritual foundation of all our traditions, ever reminding us to place principles before personalities.

motion," never seeking to gain national recognition through the cachet of celebrity converts or expensive media campaigns.

Even deeper, AA fellowship offers members a resource that so many citizens of the disenfranchised twentieth century search for in vain: the unconditional love traditionally offered by the family. "In a very fundamental way," says Allen Wood, formerly of the Alcoholism Council of Greater New York, "these anonymous self-help groups replicate the family. What they have to offer—and this is a powerful draw—is unconditional acceptance and love. This is particularly appealing for people who probably never had that in their lives. At the same time, an AA person can go anywhere and be accepted in an AA group. He will find that they will accept him and understand his problems, and speak his language, the language of recovery" (personal communication).

Nor does the support end when the doors of the meeting hall close for the night. AA members are exhorted to stay in touch by phone, to socialize, to come to one another's aid in times of temptation or emergency. This support is willingly given, accessible twenty-four hours a day, and—perhaps most important of all—free.

For many people, the group offers solace and a sanctuary among kindred spirits. But some find the group atmosphere coercive and even authoritarian. "I was thankful to AA in the beginning," recalls Tony, a thirty-two-year-old Irish writer living in Brooklyn's Park Slope neighborhood. "I had been a bloody alcoholic when I first started going to AA, and I felt proud of myself after I took the oath and kept to it." A series of hair-raising drinking sprees, including a careening weeklong bout that precipitated a street-corner blackout, had led him to AA.

After a year and a half of abstinence, Tony went drinking one night with friends and found that he enjoyed it but felt in no way tempted to resume his serious courtship with the bottle. A lot had happened to him in the eighteen months since joining AA: he had enjoyed his first success as a writer and had found a job that gave him some financial security; he now felt that there was too much at stake for him to let his drinking get out of control again. "But I couldn't get this idea across at the meeting," he recalls with a touch of bitterness. "Everybody treated me as if I had peddled my soul to the devil. Unless I swore off booze forever and ever, I was a lost soul."

Shortly after this confrontation, Tony left AA for good.

The Disease Concept and Personal Responsibility

Alcoholism progresses in stages, like any chronic disease, and cannot be reversed, either through physiological or psychiatric means. People who accept this notion are obliged to believe that there is "no such thing as one drink" and that any return to alcohol brings a return of alcoholism as well. "Hi, I'm Mary," the AA member, thirty-five years sober, announces at a meeting. "And I'm an alcoholic."

What carries the weight here is that the pathology model has a psychological force that is both liberating and healing; many AA newcomers find its message a major help in accomplishing their aim, which is sobriety.

Even though the disease model releases members from the guilt of having caused their own alcoholism, it does not in any way, despite what some critics claim, absolve them from the responsibility of dealing with it. Anyone who doubts this has not sat through enough AA meetings and has not watched enough members lovingly but firmly take fellow AAers to task for ducking their duties or for failing to keep their priorities in sight. In this sense, the AA credo mirrors what Jesse Jackson has repeatedly said to African Americans: "You may not be responsible for causing the problem. You *are* responsible for doing something about it." As Sheila Blume writes: "Relieving guilt feelings about having become an alcoholic does not relieve the patient of responsibility for following the treatment regimen and taking the steps necessary for recovery. In this respect alcoholism differs very little from other chronic diseases where following a diet, doing prescribed exercises, taking medication, attending therapy sessions, avoiding certain environmental hazards, etc. are the clear responsibility of the patient" (Blume, 1989, p. 77).

Perhaps the strongest position regarding alcoholism as a disease has been developed by James Milam and Katherine Ketcham in their classic book *Under the Influence* (1981). Later development of the idea is presented by Milam in "The Alcoholism Revolution" (1992). In essence, Milam argues that while over one hundred million people imbibe alcohol in the United States, only about 10 percent of them are potential alcoholics—people who have a physiologically different reaction to liquor, including an abnormal metabolism. He notes that studies have "uncovered a number of physiological differences between alcoholics and non-alcoholics [prior to developing alcoholism]. These 'predisposing factors' explain the alcoholic's vulnerability to alcohol and the onset of alcoholism" (Milam and Ketcham, 1981, p. 34).

All of the social and psychological difficulties of the alcoholic are the product of the addiction and do not exist prior to it. Milam and Ketcham propose a new biogenic paradigm and are strongly critical of the psychological and social paradigms in vogue. In fact, they argue at one point that these other approaches iatrogenically help sustain the alcoholism. There is one disclaimer: "Although psychological factors do not cause alcoholism, they can influence the alcoholic's attempts to control his drinking and his reaction to the addiction" (Milam and Ketcham, 1981, p. 34; see also Maxwell, 1984).

Critique

For all AA's popularity and influence, surprisingly scanty scientific data are available to tell us just how effective AA really is—or isn't—at getting alcoholics to stop drinking.

Stanton Peele, AA's stern and implacable critic, claims that several other alcoholism programs are actually more effective than AA but that due to AA's influence over American social policy, these alternatives are given short shrift.

Peele argues in *The Diseasing of America* (1989) that the disease model "does at least as much harm as good." For one thing, he believes that it minimizes the influence of environment and cultural forces on the problem drinker while undermining the individual's sense of personal accountability for his or her behavior. In Peele's view, calling alcoholism—and other dependencies—diseases encourages drug-dependent persons to slough off full responsibility for their condition by blaming it on the impersonal agent of a medical condition. Meanwhile, such thinking leads to a rampant "disease ideology," in which people tend increasingly to regard themselves as passive rather than active agents in their own addiction.

Especially culpable, Peele claims, is AA's evangelistic approach to recovery. "Although AA proposes a biological explanation for alcoholism," he writes, "its climate is that of nineteenth-century revivalistic Protestantism. The twelve steps in the AA credo are an obeisance to God (God is mentioned six times) and the need for taking moral inventory and for contrition" (Peele, 1989, p. 46).

The AA model of addiction, as Peele sees it, has risen to acceptance through a combination of media hype and hard sell. "The reasons for AA's success in selling the nation on its views of alcoholism include its remarkable appeal to the media," he writes. "From the founding of the National Council on Alcoholism, Marty Mann [a professional publicist] and others regularly presented the disease concept in magazine articles. NCA founders also consulted with the film industry in making motion pictures such as *The Lost Weekend* that presented the alcoholic's plight sympathetically" (Peele, 1989, p. 46).

AA itself admits that about half the persons who attend its meetings stop coming after three months or less. Of those who remain, however, 29 percent stay sober for five years or more, 37 percent remain sober from one to five years, and as many as 34 percent fall off the wagon in less than a year (*Hazelden*, 1993, p. 3).[1]

Certain drug rehabilitation clinics that employ AA principles and include AA involvement in treatment have a statistically more successful track record. The professionally run clinic at Hazelden, for example, claims that 60 percent of its clients remain sober or drug-free for at least two years after treatment (*Hazelden*, 1993, p. 3).

In Peele's estimation, AA's worst indiscretion is convincing alcoholics that they are "sick" people who have no command over (and hence no responsibility for) their addictive behavior. "The mission of temperance adherents and AA proselytizers has been to convey the belief that alcoholism is a disease," he tells us, "and that alcohol exercises an alluring but destructive power over our bodies and minds—our souls, in fact. . . . One of the most successful aspects of this sales job has been the convincing of liberal-minded Americans that it is most humane and helpful to regard drunkenness and other misbehavior as being out of people's control" (Peele, 1989, p. 258).

Certain other critiques of AA are equally unflattering. Psychiatrist and author George Vaillant (1983) performed an eight-year study of two groups of alcoholics. The first group was treated for alcoholism at an AA-based program at Cambridge Hospital in Massachusetts. The second group received no treatment at all.

Reviewing his findings, Vaillant discovered that there were no significant differences in sobriety attainment between the two groups and that alcoholics who were left to their own devices stayed approximately as drunk or as sober as graduates of the AA-based rehabilitation program (Vaillant, 1983).

In research studies such as Vaillant's that compare AA methodology with other intervention strategies (or with no intervention strategies at all), individuals are assigned to the various interventions, and attendance at AA meetings is mandated as part of the study. This is also true in situations where individuals are arrested for drunk driving and are then compelled by the courts or by their company's Employee Assistance Program to attend AA. In both cases, deleterious and unsuccessful results follow. Obviously, situations such as these, where subjects are forced into compliance, differ in a deeply qualitative way from those in which individuals willingly place themselves in a voluntary program. This important factor should always be considered when weighing the results of studies such as Vaillant's.

Another important criticism of AA comes from Jerry Dorsman. He argues that only 5 percent of Americans with serious drinking problems belong to AA. This is because "AA offers moral support based on a specific religious philosophy" and because "AA offers group therapy with a social support network. . . . Unfortunately many alcoholic drinkers feel terribly anxious in a group. These people can't function in a group unless they can drink" (Dorsman, 1994, pp. 3–4). This led Dorsman to develop a new self-help approach embodied in his book *How to Quit Drinking Without AA*.

Approaching the issue from a different perspective, Charlotte Davis Kasl, in her book *Many Roads, One Journey*, takes AA to task for, among other things, what she considers its sexist God concept, its "cultlike" environment, and the inappropriate moral pressures it places on members. In Kasl's estimation, AA (and twelve-step programs in general) focuses more on members' weaknesses than on their strengths, reinforcing a Christian theme of sin and redemption, which she considers outmoded and detrimental to ego strength development. In AA, she contends, there are no steps for "expressing love of people, having fun, celebrating life, and becoming powerful or healing the physical body" (Kasl, 1992, p. 138).

Equally detrimental to personal growth, Kasl believes, is the fact that AA maintains a closed inner-circle attitude toward the outside world and consistently fails to open itself up to self-review and self-examination. This, she believes, "teaches blind faith and often blocks people from seeing abuse in groups," producing ultimately a clannish and inflexible "us against them" mentality (Kasl, 1992, p. 230).

A Certain Critical Factor

When accused of these and the other transgressions, AA answers with the same single and unvarying response it has given inquisitors for sixty years: silence. Solemnly committed to staying out of public debates, whether they be political, religious, academic, or ideological, and choosing to attract followers by example and word of mouth rather than publicity, AA's posture says: "We're here if you need us. We think we're the best way to achieve sobriety. But you must come to us—we won't come to you."

This is not to maintain that AA fails in its mission, of course, or that it is less worthy than competing systems. Clearly, it keeps a number of its members sober for many years, and some studies suggest that its success rates are as at least as good as those of the competition.

For our purposes, the really intriguing issue is not whether Alcoholics Anonymous is ultimately the best game in town, or the worst, but that in many ways, for whatever reasons, it is viewed as the *only* game in town.

From a certain standpoint, this behavior leads us to believe that the popularity of AA involves certain critical factors that go beyond drinking and perhaps even beyond addiction itself.

Spirituality or Religion

Some scholars believe that AA has achieved its success by fulfilling a fundamental human need for spiritual belonging and fellowship that many signs indicate is part of the psychic blueprint of the human species.

AA is a secular movement with strong religious overtones that parallel, if not exactly imitate, the pietistic foundations of the Christian church. These qualities include AA's own version of original sin (one is born with a weakness for alcohol), a sacred credo and law (the twelve steps and the Twelve Traditions), a congregation (meetings), a litany (slogans), confession (the "drunkalogue"), conversion (quitting drinking and coming to AA), the devil (alcohol), sin and temptation (drinking), scripture (the *Big Book*), God (one's Higher Power), founders and prophets (Bill and Dr. Bob), a hagiology (Lois, Dr. Silkworth, John D. Rockefeller, Reverend Tunks), hell (drunkenness), heaven (sobriety), prayer (both the serenity[2] and private kind), faith (belief in the healing power of AA fellowship), and redemption (recovery). It also propounds a set of moral and behavioral prescriptions that, as in any religion, members are obliged to follow for the rest of their lives.

AA allows one to start life afresh, to be born again. One is not responsible for original sin, but one is responsible for one's own salvation. Likewise, one is not responsible for being an alcoholic, but one is responsible for one's own recovery. Twelve-step groups encourage people to interpret the notion of God or a Higher Power in whatever way they feel comfortable. But even though the approach is strongly nonsectarian, it is hard to see how these notions could be interpreted in a way that could be called nonreligious.

In counterresponse to the religious overtones, which put off many people, has arisen an organization called Rational Recovery, directed toward serving people with an alcohol problem who desire an approach different from AA's. However, Rational Recovery is not simply AA minus the religion. Its principles are almost diametrically opposite those of AA: opposing the powerlessness concept, advocating the use of will, providing a professional support structure, and so on. It does not require a lifelong recovery process and does not include the multifaceted community-building infrastructure characteristic of AA.

A related criticism is that AA is a cult. Apart from some emphasis on ritual, this criticism seems wholly inappropriate. Cults typically have gurus, rely on powerful mind control techniques, and are concerned with financial benefits. AA emphasizes anonymity, views leaders as trusted servants, and refuses large contributions. Compare this model to Scientology, Jonestown, or Synanon, fairly well known cults or cultlike organizations (see Hassen, 1989).

Recovery Therapy and the Commercialization of Self-Help Principles

While AA has remained steadfastly noncommercial as well as non-affiliated through the decades, a parallel recovery movement, grounded in AA principles but essentially entrepreneurial in nature, has grown up in AA's backyard.

For many people, this trend reflects a disturbing development that subverts the ideals on which what we might call "selfless self-help" was originally founded.

To comprehend the full meaning of these objections—and to discover how accurate they really are—we must take a close look at both the form and the content of the recovery movement as it exists today in the United States.

When we speak of the present-day recovery movement, we speak of two variations on a theme. *Twelve-step recovery* is recovery that takes place in a standard twelve-step program whose meetings are open to the public, not for profit, unaffiliated with any business or organization, and free of charge. *Recovery therapy* is recovery that occurs in a for-hire professional psychotherapeutic setting, usually a center, that operates, to varying degrees, on the twelve-step principles invented by AA.[3]

Generally speaking, recovery centers court the same problem populations that self-help groups administer to, from compulsive eaters to drug addicts. Drawing on a combination of self-help and professional support, these centers hire recovering twelve-steppers to fill key jobs, hand out twelve-step literature, and train their staffs in twelve-step principles. Patients may take part in AA group meetings held at the centers themselves, and they are encouraged to join groups in their own communities as well.

Accompanying this rise of professional recovery centers is a self-help communications industry that has set off a multimedia boomlet in several segments of the business community, including publishing, TV, and the novelty business. Products include books, magazines (*Changes* is one), posters, calendars, bumper stickers, buttons, computer programs, audiotapes, videocassettes, and a variety store's worth of commercial artifacts, from message coffee mugs to twenty-year medallions in Hebrew or Portuguese. Riding in on the same coattails, moreover, is a pantheon of recovery-oriented gurus, including John Bradshaw and Claudia Black, whose faces have been iconized on daytime talk shows and on the covers of best-sellers.

Yet while they borrow unabashedly from AA's twelve-step philosophy and methodology, knowing, no doubt, that AA's policy of nonaffiliation eliminates the possibility of messy legal complications, these personalities and institutions have at the same time unanimously rejected AA's disavowal of money and publicity. Some observers claim that this commercialization makes no difference as long as the healing message itself reaches people. Others argue that when the message is passed through the filter of charismatic personality and personal profit, it comes out debased and ineffectual, if not entirely squandered.

Recovery Therapy Methodology

To get in touch with the roots of their troubled histories, recovery therapy patients are encouraged to confront and reenact their childhood shocks and suffering, along with the shame, abuse, denial of feelings, and codependency that resulted. They accomplish this through a variety of techniques: role playing, psychodrama, visual imagery, group therapy, and verbal catharsis. Particular attention is paid to exposing and attacking the addictive logic ("stinking thinking") that is so characteristic of the addict's mind-set.

Part and parcel of recovery therapy is the need to deal holistically with addiction, which means, among other things, dealing with the family as well as the addict. Recovery therapy maintains three precepts: (1) addiction affects not only the addict but his or her entire familial grouping; (2) families are prone to denial and overdependency, just like the addict; and (3) to cope with the desperate reality of having an addict in their midst, family members often pursue enabling behaviors that are counterproductive to recovery. For example, they may protect the addict from the consequences of his or her destructive behavior or may expend enormous energy in keeping up the illusion of normalcy to the outside world.

Al-Anon, an AA offshoot formed in 1951, was founded to help families of addicts deal with such problems. Today its groups are a standard feature at rehabilitation centers throughout the country.

The therapeutic techniques used by recovery therapy centers are not practiced in AA meetings. AA's approach is behavioral rather than psychotherapeutic, concentrating on changing nonadaptive life habits and reconditioning present-day behavior patterns rather than delving into a member's psychological past. Like the Buddhists, who when asked whether or not God exists, reply, "If your house is burning down, first escape; then find out who set the fire," AA concentrates on escaping from alcoholism rather than analyzing the roots of the problem.

Although these systems seem to have much in common, one issue prevents their ever being best friends—that perennial bugaboo of the human resources field, the money question.

Recovery Therapy: Pros and Cons

It is difficult to ignore the gnawing money question, just as it is difficult to avoid taking potshots at the commercialization of AA's principles, at the jet-set recovery centers and "One Day at a Time" key chains.

In the process of coining clever phrases about such tawdry commercialism, however, one is apt to throw out the baby with the bath water, overlooking the critical fact that while recovery therapy does to some extent pander to Mammon, it nonetheless offers powerful methods and ideas that make it a considerably more humane and holistic approach to mental health than is generally offered by pure professionalism.

Why? Let us take inventory.

To begin, a more equal, one-to-one relationship is established in recovery therapy between patients and therapists; this, rather than the implicit "I'm OK, you're not OK" equation of patient-on-the-couch psychiatric care.

Because recovery therapists have struggled with a substance abuse or dysfunctional family problem themselves, they can share the pain of this encounter with patients along with the knowledge gained from enduring it. This mutual bond between patient and therapist, many people believe, makes a recovery therapist substantially more qualified to advise patients than an uninvolved, never-addicted professional. Indeed, most recovery therapists are in lifetime recovery mode and are usually members of a twelve-step group. Famous twelve-step advocates such as John Bradshaw make no attempt to hide their indulgent past or the fact that they are recovering alcoholics. Indeed, they use their former addiction to great psychological advantage in establishing rapport with like-minded audiences. Many best-selling pop psychologists, including Melanie Beattie, Terence Gorski, and Abraham Twerski, have written self-help books with a decidedly confessional twist.

This two-way relationship between twelve-step philosophy and recovery therapy renders special power to each. Twelve-step groups gain support from mental health professionals; recovery therapy extends its reach into the daily lives of clients via their involvement in self-help groups. Such mutual linking represents the most advanced partnership and integration of self-help and professional practice currently at work in the United States today.

Recovery Therapy and the Addiction Craze

Although there are innumerable responses to the merger of free self-help and pay-as-you-go professionalism, a majority of critics rate as the most disturbing aspects of this uneasy alliance a lessening of the spiritual commitment inherent in the twelve-step approach and a distancing of recovery groups from the community, with a concomitantly reduced interest in advocacy and social change. As one twelve-stepper put it: "When you sell your help services at the supermarket, you automatically shut things off from both directions: you stop being personally spiritual, and you stop being socially helpful."

There lies the real danger, critics claim, in a shift from the non-commercial to the overtly commercial, from the community-based to the me-based. Such melding of recovery therapy with the twelve-step method is, they claim, causing the entire self-help movement to become professionalized, therapized, and spiritually devitalized. In the process, we are witnessing the ascendancy of the self-help addict, the middle-class malcontent seeking diversion from malaise in yet one more fashionable new victim-oriented form of therapy. In short, they warn, by grafting a professional, for-profit limb onto the tree of self-help, a hybrid horror is spawned that distorts and then destroys the original idea of community-based, democratic, free, mutual self-help.

Undoubtedly, certain elements of this criticism are valid, for certainly a movement as large as recovery therapy will attract persons with less than admirable motives. On a more specific level, however, critics who fear that we are becoming a nation of self-help addicts often fail to understand the true meaning of addiction itself, the essence of which is a physical and psychological dependency on mood-altering substances or activities that relieve problems and pain, accompanied by a denial of the harmful effects of this dependency.

Though it is, of course, possible for an individual to overuse any activity, including a twelve-step program, there is an important distinction to be made here between doing something with intensity and doing it from irresistible compulsion.

In most cases—and this is important to emphasize—commitment to a twelve-step group, be it a self-help or center-based program, is in itself a sign that participants have begun to overcome the denial and resistance that were among the hallmarks of their addiction in the first place. The fact that twelve-steppers busy themselves frantically with group involvement does not necessarily mean they are "addicted" to their group, any more than people who consistently attend a church or community center are "addicted" to the purposeful and wholesome activities that take place there each day.

Moreover, the constant and perhaps overzealous use of group interaction to confront neurotic tendencies and unearth self-destructive feelings is a specific *against* addiction, not an encouragement of it. Such activities cannot by any stretch of the imagination be placed in the same category as substance dependency. Indeed, to insist that intense involvement with a twelve-step organization is the same as trading one addiction for another is much like mistaking the medicine for the disease.

In some ways, it is true, society's present preoccupation with addiction reflects the fact that many Americans feel lost and out of control. This condition can in turn be viewed as an inevitable consequence of our high-expectation, success-at-any-costs consumer culture.

Recovery therapy's response to this creeping national anomie is to place the burden of guilt on the family. According to writers like John Bradshaw, over 90 percent of American families are dysfunctional; this means, in turn, that nurturing and proper role modeling, so much part of any healthy family dynamic, have gone awry in a majority of American homes.

Perhaps, as some critics maintain, this dysfunctional model has been oversold to the public, and the family has received a larger share of the blame than it deserves. Though there is probably some truth to this assertion, it must nonetheless be acknowledged that the list of problems that beset the family is a long and dangerous one today and that under the circumstances, a bit of exaggeration may be necessary to make the point. Perhaps it has even become necessary, as they say in this age of media overkill, to poke the American public in the eye with a rafter to get its attention.

As far as the list of problems goes, moreover—child abuse and spouse abuse, incest, juvenile delinquency, drug addiction, alcoholism, suicide, violence, crime, alienation, divorce—it is necessary only to say that the unchecked spread of these afflictions in America is now apparent to just about everyone and that the inevitable result of this destructive trajectory is a weakening of the psychic foundations that make us all human and sane.

So even though it is a seller's market today for recovery therapists and the centers and therapists who deal with our national
problems are often overtly profit oriented, it is also evident that
recovery therapy programs have helped innumerable Americans
come to terms with abuses that are undermining our social system
and that in many cases, these programs have helped patients who
might otherwise have destroyed themselves.

At its best, therefore, recovery therapy brings society's calami-
tous family and personal secrets into the light of day, forcing us to
look at ourselves and our mores and to come to terms with certain
terrible realities that several decades ago were unmentionable and
hence went untreated.

Concurrently, recovery therapy has forced people to understand
that upbringing does indeed shape personality and that the manipulation and withholding of love so characteristic of dysfunctional
families truly warps a person. In the process, patients learn that it
is possible to examine their childhood via standard recovery therapy techniques, see what went wrong, forgive their transgressors,
and heal in the process. Once armed with this understanding, moreover, people carry these lessons back to their own family circle
where, it is hoped, they will be able to avoid making the same mis-
takes with their own children.

These benefits are powerful forces, and their influence should
not be minimized. Recovery therapy has influenced the twelve-step
movement itself.

This influence may be threatening because the recovery therapist is not simply another group member but, like it or not, a potential mentor as well. An element of professionalism thus creeps in
with the tutelary presence of the therapist, diluting the pure democracy of the twelve-step group.

Yet recovery therapists add a new dimension via a more sophisticated and systematic approach to addiction treatment, coupled
with the infusion of creative new therapeutic methods developed over the past decade in the human laboratories of recovery
centers.

There is then certainly no doubt that by remaining unaffiliated and noncommercial, AA has kept itself above the temptations of empire building. But it has paid a price for this resistance, many believe, by becoming insular and deaf to the music of innovative new ideas.

At the same time, the twelve-step model's success rate rests on a highly efficacious method of help-giving, a nonbureaucratic organizational model, an accent on large-scale personality transformation, and a deep commitment to helping people, especially other addicts.

In addition, AA relies on general self-help principles, most of which they invented: intermember support given at any time of day or night, free services and activities, open exchange of mutual experiences, sponsorship, reciprocity and mutual aid (as the saying goes, "I alone can do it, but I cannot do it alone"), a democratic collectivity, and a universal goal of personal empowerment.

Meanwhile, recent borrowings from AA doctrine and the use of twelve-step principles in commercial recovery centers have, in the eyes of some critics, watered down the essential self-help message. Yet despite their sometimes mercenary orientation, professional recovery centers have done much to bring twelve-step truths to public awareness and to awaken literally millions of people to the social and familial problems that beset us on all fronts.

These real benefits may be open to criticisms from many directions, it is true. But by and large, the observable and apparently positive influence that AA and other twelve-step programs have exerted on addiction problems in the United States and elsewhere suggest that they are a major source of social change in today's world.

Although our major concern in this chapter has been the implications of the twelve-step model for the self-help movement in general, it may be useful to turn directly to its application for alcoholics in general. Some ten million people in the United States are believed to have a drinking problem. There are currently about one million members of AA, and AA itself indicates that only ten of those who join remain in the program for more than three years. Clearly, then, despite its image of success, AA fails to help the vast majority of alcoholics. A number of reasons are offered to explain this phenomenon, including the quasi-religious dimension and the fact that many people may not be responsive to a group approach. We would add the distinction indicated in Chapter One between the two levels of addiction. People with a deep, complex addiction will need AA or something similar. They require a powerful counterforce to produce a personality transformation or a value transformation. Here the spiritual dimensions of AA are relevant.

For people with simple addiction, many other options appear possible, including books such as Dorsman's *How to Quit Drinking Without AA* (1994).

It may in fact be, as AA critics argue, that alcoholism is not a disease; that a number of committed AA members are not, after all, true alcoholics; and that a lifetime of commitment to this movement is ultimately counterproductive. At the same time, the twelve-step model derives much of its power from these very notions, and many people feel that in the long run, the effort is worthwhile, especially for the following reasons:

1. Through its techniques and group dynamic, AA develops a rock-hard sense of community and identity among its membership. The AA ethos makes members feel part of a network of friends who understand one another and speak the same language. For some, it provides an atmosphere of unconditional love.

2. Many members believe that involvement in AA has contributed to their personal transformation and has given them a new sense of freedom, usefulness, and serenity. Psychiatrically, the mental health of these persons has been improved. In the idiom of AA, these people have achieved a spiritual

conversion and now see themselves as integral parts of a mystical fellowship far greater and bigger than themselves.

3. AA members achieve more than simple abstinence from their involvement in groups. They do not simply become "dry drunks," craving a lost high and a last drink, as many addicts in abstinence-based programs do. Rather, the recovery process they experience, lifelong or not, brings genuine sobriety plus an increased sense of self-esteem and a meaningful philosophy of life.

Conclusion

AA relies on the general self-help principles: concrete help at any time at no cost, the understanding that derives from similar personal experience, the function of modeling ("I did it—so can you"), reciprocity (mutual aid), the power of the group ("I alone can do it, but I cannot do it alone"), the helper therapy principle ("helping helps"), and empowerment (the beneficial effects of having control over your own condition or problems).

In other words, for the dedicated member, AA is a system complete in itself, a social, psychological, philosophical, and spiritual way to fulfillment. This fact, among the many others discussed in this chapter, explains why AA-based twelve-step ideas have become popular so rapidly over the past several decades and why members feel such a deep and enduring commitment, the likes of which is rarely found in other areas of endeavor today.

In essence, the appeal of AA resides in its integration of a variety of elements, some of which may seem contradictory: a highly structured democratic organizational model combined with a ritualistic adherence to twelve programmatic steps; an acceptance of powerlessness together with strong demands for active responsibility and a commitment to change; an emphasis on spirituality and an opposition to religious dogma together with deeply enmeshed religious overtones; an accent on time-tested values (caring, community, giving) along with a modern, almost New Age openness and acceptance; and a sickness model that, while not allowing for cure, promotes control and long-term recovery. Add to this the emphasis on decommercialization, anonymity (in contrast to charismatic leadership), an antithesis to politics, a vast helping infrastructure, and a well-developed explanation for the cause of the problem and an intervention strategy for its control.

4

. . . .

Self-Help and the New Health Agenda

When we talk about health care reform in the United States, we must put it into a historical context. Health concerns have changed in the past century, yet the resources we bring to health care deal primarily, albeit effectively, with the health problems of a different era. To think about health care reform today, we need to address the following question: What resources are appropriate to current health concerns? The answers are not always obvious.

In earlier centuries, the health-related fears of individuals and nations alike were focused on acute contagious diseases. Smallpox, diphtheria, tuberculosis, cholera, pneumonia, typhoid, influenza—these were our great-grandparents' nightmares and the cause of 80 percent of deaths among people over age sixty and under age ten.

In the present era, of course, improved sanitation and housing, better diet, immunizations, antibiotics, surgery, and modern health care practices have caused the longevity curve in the industrialized world to sweep dramatically upward. Seldom do we now hear of children succumbing to bacteria-borne ailments; seldom do we read of flu epidemics decimating whole populations; seldom do we have friends—other than those with AIDS—who die from acute diseases before their thirtieth birthday, or their fortieth, or their fiftieth.

Indeed, as science labors to improve standards of living, it is concurrently—and ironically—employed in the development of a technology that produces new and previously undreamed-of sources of human illness and destruction: air pollution; contamination of farmland, food, and water; uncontrolled population expansion; global warming; mass weapons of war; dying forests and seas; plus all the other apocalyptic scenarios, real and imagined, that have come to haunt the modern sensibility.

Longevity thus comes at a high price: in this case not only the contamination of our habitat but also an assortment of long-term, progressive physical and mental ailments that often take years to express their full symptomology and that disable us—or kill us—by degrees. We simply die a little later now, and slowly.

Diabetes, cancer, heart disorders, hypertension, asthma, arthritis, emphysema, and assorted mental ailments are a few of the ills that are endemic to Western industrialized society, diseases that were of far less concern in centuries past and apparently thrive best in a world where people live more than sixty-five years.

Approximately 50 percent of the American population now suffers from some form of slow-developing, insidious illness (Levin, Katz, and Holtz, 1976). In the physician's office, over 70 percent of all visitors come for help with long-term sickness. The top causes of mortality in the United States are consistently heart disorders, cancer, cerebrovascular ailments, and various pulmonary problems such as emphysema, all of them progressive degenerative diseases.

In other words, over the course of the twentieth century, we have seen a dramatic shift in health problems from acute disorders to chronic ones. As we now think about health care reform, it is critical that we recognize the shifting health problems we face and bring to them the appropriate health care resources.

Self-Help Health Groups: Characteristics and Growth

Over the past forty years, mutual aid groups in the health field have evolved along several distinct lines to meet the needs not only of chronic patients but also of patients (and the families of patients) suffering from almost every disease, disability, mental problem, and addiction imaginable. Indeed, a degree of specialization has arisen among health-oriented groups that rivals that found in the field of medicine itself. Here is a brief sampling of these groups (for further details, see Madara and White, 1992); notice how problem-specific or population-specific most of them are.

Addiction

Anesthetists in Recovery

Chapter Nine Group of Hollywood

Chemically Dependent Anonymous

Intercongregational Alcoholism Program (ICAP)

International Doctors in AA

International Pharmacists Anonymous

Overcomers Outreach, Inc.

Social Workers Helping Social Workers

AIDS

Body Positive of New York

Family Centered HIV Project

Gay Men's Health Crisis

National Association of People with AIDS

Anemia

Aplastic Anemia Foundation of America

Cooley's Anemia Foundation

Fanconi's Anemia Support Group

National Association for Sickle Cell Disease

Ankylosing Spondylitis

Ankylosing Spondylitis Association

Apnea

Awake Network

Arachnoiditis

Arachnoiditis Information and Support Network

Arnold-Chiari Malformation

Arnold-Chiari Family Network

Arteriovenous Malformation

AVM Support Group

Arthrogryposis

Avenues: A National Support Group for Arthrogryposis

Ataxia

National Ataxia Foundation

Have you ever hear of arthrogryposis? How about arachnoiditis? Most people haven't. Yet for people suffering from incessant and excruciating contracture of the joints (arthrogryposis) or from the insidious destruction of the pia mater of the brain (arachnoiditis), such diseases are a real and terrifying daily presence. For many years, sufferers of these and other ailments, both common and rare, received minimal attention and support. So they took the bull by the horns and began to sponsor their own advocacy.

Our listing is, of course, only a smattering of groups under A. There are dozens more under that letter and hundreds of others down the alphabet, from the American Carpal Tunnel Syndrome Association to the Spina Bifida Association of America, from the Blinded Veterans Association to the Tardive Dyskinesia National Association, from the American Hirschsprung's Disease Association to Y-ME National Organization for Breast Cancer Information and Support.

Gratifyingly diverse, these groups cater to certain well-defined memberships, including the following:

1. *Patients actively suffering from a chronic disease*. Patient-oriented organizations such as the American Lupus Society and the Women's Midlife and Menopause Group exist primarily to assist persons suffering from an ongoing health problem or disorder. Members attend group meetings on a regular basis to exchange ideas with other patients, vent their frustrations, discuss current research and relevant medical issues, and generally become better educated in their field of medical concern.

2. *Patient rehabilitation*. Organizations such as the Stroke Clubs, the National Burn Victim Foundation, the American Amputee Foundation, and the Coronary Club help patients convalesce after an operation, accident, or major illness.

The National Burn Victim Foundation, for example, provides educational programs and mental health services for burn victims in their posthospital period of adjustment. The Stroke Club furnishes stroke patients with mutual support plus social and recreational activities.

Such services are often consumer-initiated and are designed to help patients get back on their feet and adapt to altered life circumstances. Indeed, many major health organizations, such as the American Cancer Society and the American Heart Association, are now sponsoring their own self-help clubs as a means of main-streaming members back into society after undergoing medical trauma.

3. *Bereavement and the terminally ill*. These organizations cater to the specialized needs of persons suffering from a terminal ailment or of the families of the dying or recently deceased. The After AIDS Bereavement Support Group provides, in its own words, "a place of comfort, hope, and strength to anyone who has lost a loved one to AIDS."

With a somewhat different slant, the ALS Association dedicates its efforts to enhancing the quality of life that remains to persons suffering from amyotrophic lateral sclerosis (Lou Gehrig's disease) and to sponsoring research in this area. Organizations such as Alive Alone, Inc.; the Huntington Disease Society of America; Children of Aging Parents; and the National Association of People with AIDS work along similar lines.

4. *Family and friends of patients suffering from a health related problem*. A separate category of groups exists for spouses, parents, children, lovers, caregivers, and friends of the patient. Perhaps the best known is Al-Anon, the Alcoholics Anonymous spin-off group that caters to the spouses of members, and Alateen, an organization for the teenage children of alcoholics. There are hundreds of other groups that concern themselves with the needs of family and friends, some of which are intensely advocative and political. The largest of these tend to be parental organizations that have pioneered major breakthroughs in the fields of education and care for disabled children by means of group influence, lobbying, and litigation.

5. *Recovering addicts*. Though not always medically related, addiction control groups are classified under the health care rubric, and for good reason. Most addictions, after all, are harmful to the body as well as the soul.

The highest-profile addiction control group in America today is, of course, Alcoholics Anonymous, followed by Narcotics Anonymous, Gamblers Anonymous, and many others.

The Rapid Rise of Medical Self-Care

Certain medically oriented self-help groups have been in existence longer than most people suppose. The International Laryngectomee Association was founded in 1952, Mended Hearts and the Dysautonomia Foundation in 1951, the National Hemophilia Foundation in 1948, and the Paralyzed Veterans Association in 1946. The need has clearly been with us for years.

And yet, when reading down a list of health-oriented self-help associations, it becomes apparent that most of these groups and affiliations, especially those dedicated to rare diseases or political advocacy, came into existence after 1975. Most were established during the 1980s—not a very long time ago. And that is surprising when we consider that a mutual aid group presently exists for every disease listed by the World Health Organization. That means that the incredibly large number of physical and mental health–related self-help organizations were founded in the past two decades.

Why, we must ask, has this phenomenon arisen so recently, and with such dramatic, even desperate speed? Mental illness has been with us for a long time, surely. So have heart attacks, arthritis, amputations, narcotic addiction, and most of the other ills that mutual aid groups have been founded to address. Presumably, the symptoms and anxieties that accompany these disorders have not changed a great deal through the years.

Why Now?

The reasons for the boom in medical self-help are many. Let us take them one at a time, seeing how in the process their sum influence has shaped and altered the health care perspective shared by millions of Americans today.

Crisis and Change in Attitudes Toward Doctors

For the first half of the twentieth century, it was an axiom that medical science was solving the world's "disease problem" once and for all and that, with antibiotics and surgery leading the charge, we were rampaging up the hill of the future into a sickness-free, germ-free world that many of us just might live to enjoy in our own lifetimes.

It was also taken for granted that doctors were the trusted leaders of this crusade. Most persons over fifty, in fact, still remember being brought up on the notion of infinite medical advancement, with the doctor-scientist hailed as a kind of secular savior.

But the years passed, and progress was slow. In fact, people seemed to be just as sick as ever. The old virulent diseases were disappearing from the world, it was true, but new and vicious diseases seemed to be replacing them just as quickly. The names and terms on the medical scorecard were different now, but no one felt much better for it.

Thus slowly, inexorably, attitudes changed.

Many people began to feel that science might not deliver on its utopian promises and that within the medical establishment, a new breed of practitioner was entering the ranks more concerned with financial profit than with humanitarian service. Health care shifted from the traditional one-on-one doctor-patient relationship to assembly-line hospital care. When a person became sick or terminally ill, the traditional haven of home and family was no longer automatically waiting; in its place stood the brick nursing hospital and old-people's home. Health insurance became increasing expensive, largely a luxury of the wealthy or the well-employed, thus forcing lower-middle-class families who couldn't qualify for welfare to go without medical benefits of any kind.

Medicare and Medicaid were launched in President Johnson's Great Society of the 1960s to stem the tide. But over the decades, this experiment took a number of unexpected turns, and medical prices doubled, tripled, quintupled. Concurrently, legal definitions of malpractice broadened, and physicians found themselves pressed to the wall and even driven from the profession by excessive litigation. The whole fabric of traditional medicine seemed to be coming unraveled, and in the process its lofty rank as a calling was somehow lost in the shuffle.

Today, attitudes toward physicians have become cynical and even distrustful. At a meeting of the Endometriosis Association, for example, women readily denounce doctors as "that quack" or "that bastard" for treating them not as a person but as a disease (and sometimes the wrong disease at that). Victims of disease may have always been this dissatisfied, but never before have they had an Endometriosis Association, a Lupus Foundation, a Self-Help for the Hard of Hearing—thousands of organizations, in fact, where people band together to compare notes, disseminate the latest research findings, and demand their rights.

Meanwhile, high-tech lab tests and sophisticated medical machinery began to supersede intuitive diagnostic skills among practitioners. Soon this technology became mandatory both for diagnosis and treatment, placing physicians at yet one more remove from their patients. The price tag that came with this brave new technology meant, of course, that medical office and hospital overhead was greater than ever before, and the costs were passed down the buying chain to the lowest link, the patient.

Finally, as a rubber-band effect of these and myriad other glitches in the health system and as a reaction to the fact that the individual patient, the person for whom the entire system was ostensibly created, seemed to have become the low person on the medical totem pole, a grassroots response led by the women's movement sprang up in the late 1960s to champion a wide range of reforms and concerns.

These reforms introduced new terms and concepts into the American vocabulary: empowerment, prevention, self-help and self-care, patients' rights, consumer advocacy and political activism, demystification of medical knowledge, a willingness to investigate alternative medicines, increased sharing of information between doctor and patients and among patients themselves, and the awarding of patients a more active voice in their own medical treatment.

Insufficient Health Care Resources

There are an estimated thirty-two million people with arthritis in the United States, ten million suffering from alcoholism, eleven million with diabetes, four million addicted to narcotic drugs, and millions of others who require attention for various physical and mental ailments. In total, more than a third of the entire population needs ongoing health care.

People suffering from arthritis can be seen as thirty-two million problems, of course. Or they can instead be viewed as thirty-two million potential helpers, caregivers, and arthritis experts. Through self-help, we can work to turn problems into solutions—in this case, transforming consumers of health care into providers of it as well.

The present ratio of health care resources to patients is low and becoming lower every year. There are not enough medical resources to go around. To cope with this scarcity, more and more people turn to the inexpensive, readily available resources found in their community: others who are struggling with the same problem. If we are going to bring the ratio of problems to resources into some sort of balance, it is hard to see how we can do so without a much greater self-help component.

Increased Interest in Alternative Medicines

One of the healing practices that receives the most attention is a traditional Chinese method whereby metal needles are inserted into various points on a patient's body (including highly sensitive areas such as the eyelids and genitals). The point of this technique is presumably to release healing energies into the patient's system so that energy blockages can be removed and the patient's body allowed to heal itself.

Today, of course, acupuncture is a credible form of nonconventional medicine, and the notion of creating conditions in a patient's system that allow the body to heal itself is the foundation on which most forms of natural medicine are based.

Many other nonconventional modalities have likewise become popular in recent decades and are, to varying degrees, practiced by millions of people every year, both as a supplement to allopathic medicine and as a substitute. The theory and reputed healing powers of these systems are controversial, and persons making an excursion into these waters are cautioned that they will have to kiss a lot of frogs before they meet a prince. "Anyone venturing into the world of alternative medicine," warned *Consumer Reports,* "is likely to find it as frustrating to explore as it is enticing. This is a field that encompasses vastly different treatments. It's a field whose practitioners range from sober academic physicians to entrepreneurial faith healers. And it's a field where there are still too few careful scientific studies, and where investigators haven't even agreed on what rules of evidence should apply" ("Alternative Medicine," 1994, p. 51).

Under the natural-medicine umbrella, for example, one finds the science of homeopathy, a standard and respected form of medicine during the nineteenth century that is today struggling to regain its former standing. Better known is herbalism, which in minor ways (healing teas, herbal elixirs) is entering the mainstream and, as pharmaceutical companies continue to develop high-profile drugs based on healing properties of plants that have been used by folk doctors and herbalists for centuries, is becoming the focus of much scientific research. Chiropractic, perennial whipping boy of the American Medical Association, continues to attract adherents across the country and to flout the attempts of medical orthodoxy to discredit it.

Other popular varieties of alternative healing, some effective, some marginal, some outright quackery, include reflexology, polarity therapy, massage, relaxation techniques, water therapy, channeling for health, biofeedback, psychic and faith healing, megavitamin treatment, hypnosis, autohypnosis, art therapy, music therapy, radionics, energy healing, acupressure, macrobiotics, tai chi, yoga, and chi gung, all of them practiced by people who no longer trust fully in the healing promises of conventional medicine—or simply cannot afford the costs. Each year it is estimated that $14 billion is paid out of pocket by Americans for nonallopathic medical treatments. A recent study found that one-third of Americans surveyed have used at least one unconventional therapy in the past year (Eisenberg, 1993). Most doctors do not know that their patients combine alternative therapy with their prescribed treatment.

As we have seen, the majority of health concerns in modern technological society no longer stem from acute illnesses, in which a doctor plays a crucial part, but from chronic diseases, where the doctor's role is occasional and patients have frequent opportunity to become involved in their own daily care. This is particularly relevant in light of the fact that all ten ailments most commonly referred to alternative therapies happen to be chronic: back problems, anxiety, headaches, insomnia, depression, fatigue, arthritis, high blood pressure, digestive problems, and allergies. In the current climate of consumer advocacy, it is probably no accident that alternative medicine's neat fit into the consumer movement makes it an attractive option for Americans. Alternative medicine is cheaper than conventional medicine or even free; it is exotic, trendy, hip, New Age, interesting, and instantly self-empowering; it is chronic-disease-oriented; it usually offers a form of intimate, one-on-one personal care from a practitioner (as opposed to the hurried, impersonal quality of most visits with an M.D.); it can in many cases be practiced on one's own without a doctor (exercise, diet, acupressure); and it dovetails with the body-oriented self-concern of American consumers, a late variant of the me-oriented 1980s, that encourages do-it-yourself forms of health care such as diet, nutrition, vitamin therapy, weight reduction, and exercise.

Within the field of nonconventional healing systems, moreover, there is a division between the externally imposed, structured forms of alternate medicine that involve a doctor, a schedule, and a prescribed regimen and the self-applied forms that come closer to medical self-care per se. Into the first category fall chiropractic, homeopathy, acupuncture, herbal medicine, art and music therapy, massage, hypnosis, and all other practitioner-oriented modalities.

In contrast is the self-oriented, self-care variety, which mediates change by and through the efforts of a patient alone or by means of patients' working on an informal basis with family and friends. Acupressure, exercise, diet, water therapy, self-hypnosis, self-applied herbal medicine, visual imagery, and meditation fall into this category. We will later focus on this dichotomy as both an important distinction in the area of self-help and as a point of focus for a discussion on addiction and self-help.

A New Emphasis on Preventive Medicine

One of the medical catchwords of the 1990s is *prevention*. A person suffering from, say, hypertension is exhorted to take his or her medication and visit the doctor for regular checkups.

At the same time, many health advocates take this notion one step further: it is equally important, they argue, that persons suffering from hypertension be sparing of salt, exercise regularly, pay attention to proper nutrition, keep regular hours, stop smoking, practice forms of tension control, and actively pursue a lifestyle that eliminates the factors that cause the hypertension. In other words, advocates claim, patients must become willing to order their daily living habits in conformity with the commonsense rules of good preventive health.

The notion that the best way to deal with a disease is to prevent it from occurring in the first place is relatively new to the American health consciousness, a product, in part, of the epidemiological shift from acute to chronic diseases.

Yet while our government, quite commendably, spends billions of dollars each year on patient education and on prevention awareness policies (as do many insurance companies, having learned from experience how much less it costs to pay for health than for sickness), the medical establishment itself appears to some critics to be lagging behind.

"Though the doctor pays a lot of lip service to prevention," claims Ron Lever, leader of a New York City Parkinson's disease self-help group, "we still find that when we talk to doctors about the whys, whats, and hows of prevention, they look at us blankly. Either they don't know much about prevention, or they're not saying. That's one of the reasons we attend our group—to help each other figure out ways of preventing the problems that come with the Parkinson's territory" (spoken at Parkinson's Self-Help Meeting, November 1993).

The growing emphasis on prevention, we should affirm, is closely allied with the self-help movement in several fundamental ways.

Alcoholics who follow the precepts of AA or other recovery groups, for example, are automatically at lesser risk of developing the numerous diseases associated with alcoholism. Likewise, they are delivered from the hazards of drunk driving, alcohol-related accidents, and barroom brawls. Just as important, the psychological stress that drinking imposes on a personal level is reduced to varying degrees in the lives of recovering addicts, and hence the mental health of families and associates improves as well. All these behavioral modifications have a deterrent effect, and all therefore spare the community, state, and government untold amounts of health care money, legal fees, and social headaches.

In this light, the work of many self-help groups is preventive as well as supportive and thus contributes directly to the improvement of our national health. Typical of such groups is Mothers Against

Drunk Driving (MADD), which actively lobbies for better traffic control laws and works on several levels to educate people in the perils of drunken driving. Prevention is likewise a much discussed and frequently implemented activity among members of medically oriented self-help groups, especially support groups for specific chronic disorders such as diabetes, heart disease, and cancer where precautionary self-care techniques (such as diet, exercise, and abstinence from alcohol and tobacco) reduce both the incidence and the progression of the disease.

Finally, it is interesting to note that the preventive efforts generated by individual self-care groups have exerted a slow but steady influence on government legislation, like so many raindrops making a sea. Laws banning smoking on airplanes and in restaurants in the interest of public health are clear examples of preventive medicine and have come about at least in part as a result of pressure by advocacy groups across the country. Lobbying efforts by organizations such as MADD and Remove Intoxicated Drivers (RID) have resulted in stiffer penalties for drunken drivers. Both areas demonstrate how self-help advocacy can ultimately effect social policy and how thousands of single, independent, grassroots efforts add up over time to benefit the health of millions of people.

The Self-Care Movement

Frustrated by the alienation, overprofessionalization, and high cost of much traditional medical care, many people have been turning to self-care as a more community-centered and empowering approach to health.

Another factor in the rise of health-oriented self-help, one that is closely allied both to the philosophy of prevention and to the alternative medicine movement, is medical self-care.

In the past twenty years, the self-care movement has grown in quantum leaps, and today it supports a minor industry of magazines, books, phone help lines, training classes, home medical equipment, self-care organizations, and political lobbying. Its philosophy affirms that many ailments that are ordinarily treated in a physician's office can easily be dealt with at home by persons who are trained in self-care.

Self-care has thus been defined as "consumer performance of activities traditionally performed by providers." A British study reports that "some attempts at self-care and advice from others have been carried out by more than 80–90 percent of patients" before they visit a doctor, and that only "20 percent of all symptom experiences result in medical contact." Evidence indicates that 75 percent or more of health care is undertaken today without professional intervention (Levin, Katz, and Holtz, 1976, p. 85).

Though the reasons for this behavior vary, there are two main motivating factors: patients feel that their ailment is not serious enough to warrant a trip to the doctor, and patients cannot afford current medical fees.

In many senses, moreover, self-care activities overlap activities traditionally practiced by self-help and mutual aid groups. The two have many things in common: health education, training in coping skills, and the recognition of the three stages (described by Strauss two decades ago and still relevant today) required by an individual to cope with chronic illness: the ability to read signs that portend a crisis, the ability to respond to the crisis of the moment, and the ability to establish and maintain a regimen (Strauss, 1973).

Both self-care and mutual aid activities are, moreover, movements away from "medicocentrism"—health care that is medically centered—and both stress the responsibility that individuals must bear for their own well-being. As such, these movements also have much in common with the women's health movement, with its emphasis on self-determination and self-empowerment.

Basic to the concept of self-care is the study of the biological principles of health and the mastery of clinical skills necessary for care, healing, and health maintenance. Patients are trained to detect and manage common medical problems, to distinguish the common from the uncommon, and to engage in health-promoting activities. In some cases, the disorders that patients self-medicate are acute problems such as headache or minor flu for which effective home remedies and over-the-counter medications are available. All the doctor can do in such situations is suggest simple therapeutic measures that an informed medical consumer would know about already.

In other instances, the ailment may be a chronic one; and here again, after the primary diagnosis has been made by a physician and a form of treatment has been prescribed, self-maintenance supported by phone consultation and progress updates accomplish as much an office visits, thus saving the doctor time and the patient money.

Although many elements of medical practice are forbiddingly technical, advocates of self-care claim that basic paramedical techniques can be learned by anyone, even children. Indeed, many educators urge that such skills be taught as a regular part of the curriculum in grade schools and high schools and that self-care for common ailments be made a part of every young person's awareness. In the words of polio vaccine pioneer Jonas Salk, "It's for this reason that studying human nature—to see how to help people help themselves to become their own health managers—is the new challenge. Such studying of human nature has to start very early in life. Beyond reading, writing and arithmetic, we have to introduce into the educational system an understanding of biology, especially human biology. That understanding will guide us in becoming skillful in living healthy, constructive, contributing lives" (Holden, 1985, p. 70).

The New Advocacy and Empowerment Ethos

When self-help began to spread widely in this country, advocacy was a moderate priority. For example, early women's health groups were almost exclusively small support groups focused on personal issues. Emphasis was placed on increasing awareness of women's health needs, reexamination of sexual roles, and the provision of group counseling for female-oriented health problems.

Early AIDS groups were formed almost exclusively by patients, friends, and family in small peer-oriented, problem-centered groups to provide emotional support for persons enduring this terrible disease. Little attention was paid to public image or advocacy.

As time passed, however, and as group members began to feel that AIDS sufferers were being discriminated against by society and medical facilities alike and that the government was dragging its heels on AIDS research, a groundswell of angry reaction arose.

The result was that a local supportive network formed originally to administer to the sick and dying became a prominent social cause, which in turn proliferated into a national crusade. The National Association of People with AIDS was founded in 1986 to help and succor AIDS patients. Its original intent was primarily supportive. Today this organization provides phone mail and legal assistance, maintains an electronics network and a speakers bureau, and offers, in its own words, "a collective voice for health, social, and political concerns."

A number of other AIDS groups have become similarly politicized—so much so, in fact, that the AIDS movement itself, born and bred in a grassroots, self-help environment, has become one of the most active political advocacy movements in the United States.

Within a decade or so, under the influence of both the feminist movement and the growing power of consumer advocacy, the focus in these groups became broader and far more deeply social.

"One of the most important expressions of self-help is found in the feminist perspective," writes Audrey Gartner in an article for *Social Policy* magazine.

The feminist focus on health and body issues, fostered by the shared experiences of consciousness-raising groups, has broadened until today it encompasses self-help and know-your-body courses, alternative health care services, women's centers and clinics, telephone counseling, referral and information services such as WISH (Women in Self-Help) and WASH (Women's Association of Self-

Help), and a distinguished body of literature, including books (*Our Bodies, Ourselves* is the best example), pamphlets on various medical topics, and exposés. Among the self-help groups dealing with specific health issues are DES-Action, Reach to Recovery (for women who have mastectomies), and Womanpause (for older women) [Gartner, 1985, p. 25].

To this list we might add a variety of other organizations: Depression After Delivery, a help and support organization for women suffering from postpartum depression; the National Black Woman's Health Project, a group "committed to the empowerment of all women through wellness"; Por La Vida, bilingual self-help health care groups for Hispanic women; WMM (Women, Midlife & Menopause), a mutual support group for women passing through the change of life; DAWN (Disabled Women's Network), a feminist organization providing support and advocacy for women with disabilities; and many more.

"Underlying the formation of women's self-help groups," writes Gartner, "is the basic principle that health-related knowledge is not just the province of the health professionals but can be shared among all who want it. In addition, those experiencing a particular health condition provide mutual benefits and supports to others by sharing these experiences" (Gartner, 1985, p. 30).

Another inroad made by the upsurge in advocative spirit is the public recognition that domestic and neighborhood violence is not simply a social hazard and legal concern but a public health menace as well, one that must be dealt with in much the same way as we deal with sickness or addiction.

In response to this realization, a number of mutual aid groups are currently helping members cope with issues of domestic violence, child and spouse abuse, juvenile delinquency, and neighborhood crime. MAD DADS, Inc. (Men Against Destruction Defending Against Drugs), for example, is a new group aimed at preventing neighborhood drug and gang violence. Parents Anonymous is an

established network of twelve hundred peer-led, professionally facilitated groups for parents who abuse their children and who wish to
learn more effective methods of parenting. The National Organization of Victim Assistance (NOVA) offers support and advocacy for
victims of violent crimes. There are many more.

An increasingly important and informed voice has been making itself heard and needs to be more significantly recognized in
national health care reform. That voice comes not from "expert"
professionals but from people who have been through experiences
themselves (women with breast cancer, parents of murdered children, people with AIDS) and have significantly educated themselves about policy issues.

Current health problems are more responsive than traditional
acute illnesses to behavioral intervention. Even for AIDS, perhaps
the closest thing to the contagious diseases that haunted our ances-
tors, while the symptoms are ameliorated by medical intervention,
the most effective deterrents are behavioral and educational. As
movement activists have stressed, critical dimensions of the
response include mutual aid groups, self-care, and advocacy.

Violence, too, is a major epidemic and calls for innovative
behavioral response, including peer helper groups in schools and
self-help groups for victims and rehabilitated perpetrators, to say
nothing of a refocused media presentation of the issue.

The struggles over these and related issues will no doubt continue long after the current health care reform debates are over. As
we talk about reform, however, it is critical that we base it on an
understanding of how health needs have changed in the course of
the past century and the nonprofessional responses to current needs
that seem to work for millions of people.

Lifestyle, Personal Responsibility, and Health

Of the approximately 2,150,000 deaths recorded in 1990, approximately 800,000 could be traced to tobacco use (400,000 deaths),

diet or activity (300,000 deaths), or alcohol (100,000 deaths). Another 500,000 deaths involved sexual diseases and illicit drug use. These various factors were thus associated with 40 percent of all deaths in the country in one year. The proximate causes of death in the tobacco group included cancers, heart disease, stroke, low birth weight, and burns. In the poor-diet-and-activity group, deaths were caused by stroke, diabetes, and colon cancer. Lifestyle choices cannot produce immortality, but they can influence illness and delay death (Kallman, 1994).

Much has been made of the importance of lifestyle in the overall health of a group or a nation. Some theorists argue that in the final analysis, consumers can make choices about the food that they eat, the games that they play, the stress that they endure, and even the health care that they purchase. Victor Fuchs's classic statement is relevant here: "It is becoming increasingly evident that many health problems are related to individual behavior. In the absence of dramatic breakthroughs in medical science, the greatest potential for improving health is through changes in what people do and do not do for themselves" (Fuchs, 1972, p. 22).

Critics argue that much of this highly individualistic behavior is controlled by social factors—for example, the advertising of the tobacco industry, most recently focused on young people and minorities. But self-care, as it acquires an advocacy context, may enable social movements to emerge that affect health care enormously. Presently, such behavior has helped launch the antismoking movement.

The effectiveness of the antismoking movement derives from a convergence of many forces that ultimately produce an impact on lifestyle habits. These forces include major segments of the health establishment originally spearheaded by the surgeon general, the wellness movement, legislation concerned with the relation of prevention to cost effectiveness, New Age types of medical care, and the growing constituency of nonsmokers and, perhaps most zealous, ex-smokers, despite the power of the tobacco industry and lobbyists.

The point is that even though lifestyle choices are operationally individual, they may influence social movements.

Effectiveness of Self-Help

At present, methodologically rigorous research on the effectiveness of health-oriented self-help groups has not been carried out to any lengthy extent. Thomas J. Powell, director of the Center for Self-Help Research and Knowledge Dissemination at the University of Michigan, has listed some of the factors that complicate research (Powell, 1993). Among them are loosely defined samples, differences in operation and intent in group meetings (even among such established programs such as AA), flawed research designs, and differences in the interpretation of study results.

Although there remains much to learn concerning who benefits from self-help, how, and why, it appears that self-help participants do profit, to varying degrees, from the group experience. The following studies offer a typical overview of how self-help interfaces with the health care establishment in general and how it tends to benefit participants in a number of ways.

- A group of 105 men and women suffering from rheumatoid arthritis participated in a psychologist-mediated mutual support group and were studied under controlled conditions. A majority showed greater improvement in joint tenderness than patients in a similar group that did not take part in the study (Shearn and Fireman, 1985).

- A group of high-risk elderly patients with emphysema, chronic bronchitis, and asthma participated in self-help activities over a six-month period. Participants, it was learned, were less likely to be hospitalized over a period of time (20 percent versus 64 percent) than other high-risk patients. Those among the participants who were hospitalized tended to remain in the hospital for shorter periods of time than nonparticipating high-risk patients suffering from the same problem (Jensen, 1983).

- Adults who underwent surgery or bracing for treatment of scoliosis and who then participated in a peer support group demonstrated fewer psychosomatic symptoms, higher self-esteem, and a better patient-physician relationship than those in a nonparticipating group (Hinrichsen, Revenson, and Shinn, 1985).

Though their contribution to physical recovery and patient self-image appear to be high, health-related mutual aid groups are free of charge, thus reducing costs even as they improve quality of service and care.

A program known as Patient Activation developed by Keith W. Sehnert, director of Georgetown University's Center for Health Education, tutored a group of participants in the following areas of self-care and prevention: arteriosclerosis, motor vehicle accidents, cirrhosis, stroke, breast cancer, uterine cancer, and rheumatic heart disease; compliance with medical regimens; hypertension, nutrition; growth and development; common childhood illnesses; contraception, family planning, and venereal disease; medications; alcoholism; mental health and family relations; yoga; and automation in health care. The program relied heavily on decision-making protocols and algorithms. Although precise figures are difficult to come by, the self-care techniques taught in this program (which were made the basis of courses in eight other states) are estimated to have saved government and consumers hundreds of millions of dollars in health-related expenditures.

Self-help mutual support groups are a potentially cost-effective means of dealing with health issues, in terms of both prevention and intervention, especially with regard to the chronic care of long-term illness, such as in the following examples:

- Women suffering from metastasized breast cancer participated in a once-a-week, ninety-minute support group that stressed coping methods, emotional support, and the use of self-hypnosis for pain. On the average, participants survived twelve to eighteen months longer than women with no group affiliation. These findings are based on an analysis of survival time, at ten-year follow-up periods, of fifty women assigned to support groups and thirty-six women assigned to control groups (Spiegel, 1993).

- A group of women joined either a peer-led or a professional-led support group for caregivers of elderly parents. After eight weekly two-hour sessions, participants reported significant improvements in caregiving skills, compared to caregivers in a control group, who made few or no gains. Participants also reported acquiring expanded knowledge of local community resources, though no differences were reported between the two groups in terms of emotional fulfillment or reduction of caregiver-related stress (Toseland, Rossiter, and Labreque, 1989).

- Sixty men and women participated in a self-help group for laryngectomized cancer patients. Interviews revealed that participants sensed improvement in their communication and social skills as a result of taking part in the groups. Most of those interviewed also reported an absence of postsurgical depression (Richardson, 1980).

- A group of nurses working in a pediatric intensive care unit participated in a self-help support group. Participants reported that the experience improved both their morale and their communication skills. The turnover rate of nurses at the hospital who participated in these groups was also correspondingly low (Weiner and Caldwell, 1983–84).

Access

To make self-help a critical ingredient of health care reform, easy public access is a necessity. This process is best carried out by forging a link between self-help services and the formal health care establishment.

At present, a number of regional self-help clearinghouses provide medical references for consumer and information referral. Local clearinghouses have developed techniques to identify, recruit, and train self-help leaders who are culturally diverse and are pivotal in helping provide wide access to health-related services. At the same time, doctors and health care professionals themselves are, to varying degrees, becoming increasingly aware of self-help's value, and physician referral rates are on the rise, although acceptance of self-help by the medical care establishment remains sluggish.

Conclusion

We live in a world of expanding medical needs and shrinking medical resources. As a reaction to this conflict and to undermined faith in the medical establishment, a counterforce has arisen, encouraging a variety of patient empowerment notions. These include the demystification of medical knowledge, an increased openness toward alternate medical modalities, an emphasis on prevention and self-care, the enabling of the patient via advocacy and patient rights, the use of patients as resources, and a movement away from dependency on professional sources and toward a combining of professional and self-help services.

These developments will, of course, play themselves out in the arena of health care and public policy in the decades to come. Attention will be focused with special intensity on the following issues:

- How will self-help activities relate to present reimbursement practices and to a national health program
  in general?

- How will the operation of extended programs of self-
  help and self-care relate to present and future patterns
  of care, especially as regards health maintenance organizations (HMOs)?

- How will preventive and medical self-care programs fit
  in with present and future health programs?

- What part will patient education and empowerment
  play in the decades to come?

- What will the development of self-care modalities
  mean for the training and retraining of professionals
  and paraprofessional providers?

- To what extent will health care professionals recognize
  the value of self-care modalities and incorporate them
  into the overall therapeutic structure?

The struggles over these and related issues will no doubt continue in both the health and public areas, and developments in one
will affect developments in the other.

5

Self-Help and Mental Health

In the very broadest sense, all self-help activities promote mental health. Whatever problem or issue is being addressed, self-help goals are mental health goals: improving the individual's sense of well-being and minimizing the negative psychosocial consequences of problems. Self-help groups also pursue their goals by psychosocial means, strengthening coping skills, providing an opportunity to vent feelings, and offering social support and a context for normalization.

Self-Help for People with Psychiatric Disorders

As users of mental health services, self-helpers whose common concern is psychiatric disorders are more likely to be designated "consumers."

Condition-specific self-help groups exist for people affected by mood and affective disorders, anxiety disorders, and substance abuse disorders. In addition, several groups address mental disorders more generally, including consumer groups that challenge the very notion of using psychiatric diagnoses to label people. Some

This chapter was written with the assistance of Susan Baird Kanaan, who conducted the interviews for it.

individuals in this category, having had negative experiences with psychiatric treatment, prefer to be called ex-patients or (treatment) survivors.

For affective disorders, the predominant national organization is the National Depressive and Manic Depressive Association (NDMDA), based in Chicago. With some 250 chapters, the NDMDA has since 1986 pursued a mixed agenda of mutual support, public information, and advocacy. In addition, the *Self-Help Sourcebook* (Madara and White, 1993) lists two twelve-step networks for people with depression. A national self-help network also exists for women experiencing postpartum depression and another for people coping with seasonal affective disorder (SAD).

In the anxiety disorders field, the largest and most visible national organization is the Anxiety Disorders Association of America (ADAA), whose members include clinicians and researchers as well as consumers. The ADAA facilitates a network of autonomous self-help groups. In addition, three national self-help networks exist for people with obsessive-compulsive disorder. As with affective disorders, the great prevalence of anxiety disorders makes possible the formation of local self-help groups in many communities, groups that may or may not have a connection to a national body. In most cases, they can be located through local self-help clearinghouses or mental health associations. One active group is AIM (Agoraphobics in Motion).

Although schizophrenia is far less prevalent than anxiety and affective disorders (the latest study estimates the lifetime incidence at well under 1 percent of the population, compared to over 11 percent for each of the others), self-help groups do exist for people coping with it. One such organization is Schizophrenics Anonymous. Schizophrenia is also a major focus of the National Alliance for the Mentally Ill (NAMI), many of whose members have close relatives with the disorder. Although no data are available, it is reasonable to assume that many members of the ex-patient and survivor groups (to be described shortly) have a diagnosis of schizophrenia because a basic tenet of these groups is opposition to forced hospitalization, which is often used with this condition.

Two national ex-patient, consumer, and survivor networks complete this brief survey of mental health self-help groups: the National Association of Psychiatric Survivors and the National Mental Health Consumers Association. These groups were especially important in the 1970s and 1980s as coordinators of nationwide networking among mental health consumers.

Although Recovery, Inc., is a long-lived mental health program with self-help elements, its unique character sets it apart. The *Self-Help Sourcebook* adds that Recovery, Inc., "offers a self-help method of will training" (Madara and White, 1992, p. 109). Designed by Chicago psychiatrist Abraham Low in 1937 "to prevent relapses in former mental patients and chronic symptoms in nervous patients" (Madara and White, 1992, p. 109), Recovery prescribes a rigid structure, an assigned text (Low's *Mental Health Through Will Training*), and the leadership of a trained layperson. Its approach focuses on behavior, emphasizing self-control and willpower. Norma Raiff has done an excellent study of Recovery, Inc. (Raiff, 1984).

For decades, Recovery was the only game in town for people with mental disorders, and it remained the predominant one. A 1957 study by the Joint Commission on Mental Illness and Health reported approximately five thousand members in forty-two organizations of mental patients, four thousand of whom were in 250 Recovery groups. A 1973 study reported fifteen thousand members in 850 groups.

Dual-Diagnosis Groups

The comorbidity between depression and anxiety disorders, on the one hand, and substance abuse, on the other, makes it necessary to take a broad view not only of mental health problems but also of the self-help approaches that are used to alleviate them. In the twelve-step and recovery world, one response to comorbidity is the dual-diagnosis group, which is becoming a common variant of the Alcoholics Anonymous approach.

For their part, many self-help groups in the mental health field have developed ways of helping members address substance abuse problems. Consumer-run programs such as drop-in centers, because of their policy of turning no one away, have many clients with substance abuse problems, although their target clientele is people with psychiatric conditions.

The twelve-step model is used by several groups that take a generic approach to mental disorders rather than focusing on a single psychiatric condition such as depression or agoraphobia. Examples are Children's and Youth Emotions Anonymous, Emotions Anonymous (with twelve hundred chapters), and Neurotics Anonymous.

In this category, a self-help group that has received considerable attention through the research of Julian Rappaport is GROW (Rappaport and others, 1985). GROW is described in the *Self-Help Sourcebook* as "a twelve-step mutual help program to provide know-how for avoiding and recovering from a breakdown." The program is notable in part for having been formed some three decades before most self-help groups in the mental health field, partly inspired by the AA example.

Rappaport describes GROW's core constituents as people "with a history of hospitalization who are now in a crisis." One hundred groups in America use its model, which emphasizes mutual support and encouragement along with the creation of a "caring and sharing community" that mediates between members and the larger community. Rappaport notes that because of the depth of its involvement in members' lives and the network of groups it sustains, GROW is more a self-help organization than a self-help group.

Self-Help for Family Members

The families of people with mental health or other problems can be said to be both "primary" and "secondary" consumers—primary in terms of their experience as caregivers and secondary in terms of their relation to the root problem borne by the person in their care. The distinction between primary and secondary becomes important when there are conflicts between the perspectives, interests, and goals of caregivers and their charges. Robert Emerick found that "the most important distinction" made by people in the mental health ex-patient movement is between primary and secondary consumer groups. Often, he says, the two are "philosophically, politically and pragmatically" antithetical (Emerick, 1989, p. 283).

Many self-helpers came to self-help in their capacity as caregivers and family members—that is, because of the physical illness, mental illness, or addiction of a family member or because of another precipitant such as bereavement. Thus many self-help organizations include a wing for family members.

In addition to activities around the precipitating condition, several self-help groups and networks exist to address the concern of caregiving. Most of these are targeted at the age group or relationship of the individual being cared for—for example, Children of Aging Parents or the Well Spouse Foundation. A dynamic new organization, the National Association of Family Caregivers (NAFC), based in the Washington, D.C., area, was formed by two caregivers (one whose husband has multiple sclerosis and the other whose mother has Alzheimer's disease) to provide support and advocacy at the national level for family caregivers of all kinds. Focusing on advocacy and education, the NAFC is growing rapidly toward its goal of connecting and speaking for the estimated seventeen million Americans—80 to 90 percent of whom are women—with major informal caregiving responsibilities. It emphasizes providing members with "actionable information" on caregiving.

One of the most powerful and effective caregivers' organizations in the country is the National Alliance for the Mentally Ill, which since its creation in the early 1980s has grown to a position of great influence in the mental health field. The typical NAMI member is a parent fifty to seventy years of age with a schizophrenic child (usually a son) aged between twenty-five and forty (*Harvard*, 1993). NAMI is decentralized, and local groups meet in members' homes. Local, state, and national levels of the organization have their own fundraising structure, newsletters, and other features.

NAMI grew out of the efforts of national leaders such as Agnes Hatfield to unite dozens of community-based groups into a single network that could speak with one voice about national policy. The rapid growth of the organization is a testament to bottom-up momentum from local communities and widespread recognition of the need for a national organization. The founding conference in September 1979 was attended by 284 people representing fifty-nine local and state self-help groups from twenty-four states and Canada. Most groups were composed of parents who had come together to obtain mutual support and to press for more humane and effective forms of treatment for their mentally ill family members.

By 1982, NAMI had 160 affiliates with eight thousand members, and the five-hundredth NAMI affiliate had been enrolled by late 1985. Once the national organization was created, this in turn stimulated the growth of more state affiliates. Alfred Katz notes that its size now threatens to undermine NAMI's grassroots character because members do not know each other personally and "local members have yet to learn politically effective ways of expressing their will to the national body" (Katz, 1993, p. 50).

In 1983, NAMI intensified its efforts to stimulate federal support for research on schizophrenia and depression. The National Alliance for Research on Schizophrenia and Depression was created in 1985, with a governing board of primary and secondary consumers and a scientific council with twenty-two prominent psychiatrists. The group's efforts have resulted in demonstrable increases in funding for research and the strong participation by NAMI representatives in such influential bodies as the National Mental Health Leadership Roundtable.

The National Alliance for the Mentally Ill has also been instrumental in maintaining funding through the budget-cutting 1980s for the Community Support Program and other social programs. Katz reports that "the national NAMI office was very active in efforts to save the Community Support Program of the [National Institute of Mental Health], to resist Social Security reviews and cuts for disabled persons, and to increase research funding" (Katz, 1993, p. 47).

NAMI is included among caregiver self-help groups because even though its members include people with psychiatric disorders, it is primarily composed of family members. They came together in response to the major shifts brought about in the 1970s and 1980s by both deinstitutionalization and new insights into brain disease and its treatment.

Self-Help for Coping with Life Crises and Transitions

This category covers nonmedical areas, including bereavement, other major life transitions, victimization, and family problems. Self-help groups are often the intervention of choice for people coping with such problems.

The *Self-Help Sourcebook* lists twenty-three national or international groups concerned with bereavement. Most of these groups are highly specific as to the cause or circumstances of death (for example, Pan American flight 103, sudden infant death syndrome, murder, suicide). One of the most general is THEOS (They Help Each Other Spiritually), with over one hundred chapters internationally that "assist widowed persons of all ages and their families to rebuild their lives through mutual self-help." Another national organization for people experiencing bereavement is Compassionate Friends, founded in 1969.

In addition to the local affiliates of national groups such as these, many communities have freestanding bereavement groups. They may be affiliated with a local hospital, church, or mental health center. One that has self-help components, using a one-to-one approach rather than groups, is Widow-to-Widow (Silverman, 1986).

Self-help groups have formed to cope with the experience of physical and sexual abuse, for victims of abuse as well as for parents of young victims. In the category of sexual abuse, incest, and rape, the *Self-Help Sourcebook* lists nine national organizations and eleven "model" groups (presented as resources for people wishing to start similar groups). Most of these abuse-related groups combine mutual support, empowerment, public awareness, and advocacy efforts. Some hold conferences, publish newsletters, and facilitate pen-pal programs. Some use the twelve steps or the Twelve Traditions developed by Alcoholics Anonymous. Reflecting its commitment to serving as a resource for new groups, the *Sourcebook* includes several entries in this section as suggested resources for people wishing to start groups (for example, for battered women).

In the crime and violence category, several national groups combine support and advocacy around the experience of crime and murder and in support of victims' rights. Parents of Murdered Children has 325 chapters and contact persons throughout the United States and Canada. One of its services is to accompany parents to court. Since 1984, the National Alliance for the Mentally Ill has maintained a forensic committee to support families of mentally ill persons in prison or in the criminal justice system.

Self-help groups also exist for offenders in the abuse and crime categories, including Batterers Anonymous, Parents Anonymous, and Convicts Anonymous. The predominance of twelve-step groups in this category indicates that the twelve-step approach is considered useful in overcoming a variety of unwanted behaviors besides substance abuse.

People coping with family issues such as adultery, divorce, custody battles, raising grandchildren, and single parenting can also turn for help to national organizations of people who "have been there." Many such organizations offer resources for finding or starting local self-help groups. Chicago-based We Saved Our Marriage ("for spouses whose marriage is affected by infidelity") has ten national affiliates and offers assistance in starting groups. Founded in 1987, Grandparents as Parents (GAP) has over two hundred groups in which members "share experiences and feelings." Omaha-based MAD DADS (Men Against Destruction Defending Against Drugs) was founded in 1989 to fight community gang- and drug-related violence by "providing family activities, community education, speaking engagements, and 'surrogate fathers' who listen to and care about street teens." This self-help group's agenda typifies the use of community action as a prime means of self-help, working toward a social goal that is regarded as personally beneficial.

One of the "granddaddies" of family-oriented self-help groups is Tough Love International, founded in 1979, with 650 groups internationally. Its core activity is parent-to-parent support for "dealing with the out-of-control behavior of a family member." The juxtaposition of Tough Love with the next listing in the *Sourcebook* illustrates the range of problems addressed by self-help. The listing, a "model" group in Kalamazoo, Michigan, is Abused Parents of America, which provides "mutual support and comfort for parents who are abused by their adult children."

Sixteen national groups are listed in the separation and divorce category of the *Sourcebook,* including groups for parents having difficulty collecting child support payments, for fathers concerned with equal custody rights, for children of separated or divorced parents, for grandparents seeking visitation rights, and for separated and divorced Catholics. In addition, there are three national groups for single parents and one for stepfamilies, the latter with more than sixty-five chapters.

There are no firm boundaries between self-help groups and other groups of citizens focused on such problems as unemployment, homelessness, tenant management, welfare rights, and crime prevention. Countless community action groups in this country work on local community issues. Some of them help members address personal concerns such as family problems, poor health, and addiction. Their broader social agendas reflect a conviction that mental health cannot be achieved without improved living conditions.

The Ex-Patient and Survivor Movement and Consumer-Run Services

The growth of self-help programs for mental health consumers began in the early 1970s, when the principles of the civil rights movement were applied to the problems of people living in mental hospitals. . . . Psychiatric patients actively sought self-determination . . . [and] freedom from domination by professional caregivers. . . . Ex-patient groups . . . founded local and national organizations (such as the Mental Patients Liberation Front), published newsletters (such as *Madness Network News*), and challenged the established system on such topics as commitment to mental hospitals, involuntary treatment, patient abuse. . . .

For persons in these groups the mutual support of others with similar experiences was just as valuable as the assertion of rights. . . . Self-help groups, drop-in centers, and other alternatives counterbalanced exclusive dependence on professional caregivers. In this way consumer-operated mental health services eventually evolved. . . . The transition was aided by the Community Support Program (CSP), a project of the National Institute of Mental Health (NIMH) in which consumers demanded and achieved influential participation. The CSP provided funding for a range of consumer operated services since the late 1970s [*Harvard*, 1992].

The world of consumer-run mental health services is far too complex to represent adequately here. Fortunately, a number of highly informative and thoughtful firsthand accounts and analyses are available (see Chamberlin, 1978; Zinman, Harp, and Budd, 1987).

The arenas of self-help activity by mental health consumers include local self-help groups, consumer involvement in state mental health programs, consumer-run services, joint research efforts, and a variety of national organizations and networks. Emerick described the "typical" mental health consumer group this way in 1989, based on his study of 104 groups: "The typical [mental patient] movement group is located in a large metropolitan area of one-quarter million or more population. The typical group is two or three years old. It operates on an annual budget of about $30,000, has a membership composed of approximately 33 people, and a leadership cohort of 3 or 4 people. We also found a concentration of movement groups in three clusters—one on the East coast, one on the West coast, and one in the upper Midwest" (Emerick, 1989, p. 298). This characterization, however, conceals wide variations among groups in size, budget, leadership, location, age, politics, and other aspects.

Ex-patient groups began to form in the 1970s as an outgrowth of the civil rights movement and a response to unacceptable treatment practices, hastening the rate of deinstitutionalization by forcing the closure of large state-operated institutions. Two networks, the National Mental Health Consumers Association and the National Association of Mental Patients (later renamed the National Association of Psychiatric Survivors), grew out of those early efforts and spearheaded national organizing to change conditions in psychiatric institutions, end discrimination, and develop alternatives to the mental health system.

These efforts were strengthened by the establishment of the Community Support Program (CSP) in 1977 by the National Institute of Mental Health. To this day, the CSP facilitates and supports the involvement of consumers in the planning, delivery, and evaluation of psychosocial services. Although its budgets have been small by federal budgetary standards, the CSP has been instrumental in helping self-helpers realize their goals of self-determination by supporting innovative community programs with a strong consumer role. The CSP has provided start-up money for model programs, encouraged service models that foster consumer empowerment, and reinforced grassroots infrastructures in every state in the nation.

The combined impact of mental health consumers and the CSP was strengthened in 1986 by two critical pieces of legislation, the Mental Health Planning Act of 1986 and the Protection and Advocacy for Mentally Ill Individuals Act, both of which required the formal involvement of consumers and family members in advisory and planning bodies for mental health services. At present, the CSP is emphasizing employment and independence.

The developments that began in the 1970s created opportunities for consumers to interact with policymakers, professionals, administrators, family members, and others from a position of strength. The resulting snowball effect is still under way: as the consumer movement has grown and become more influential, the demand for consumer-operated programs has increased.

One sphere of consumer mental health activity involves the official programs run by state departments of mental health and often partly funded by the National Institute of Mental Health. In particular, state offices of consumer liaison are a growing force today. These offices are staffed by mental health consumers who represent consumer issues to the state and assist self-help groups. The CSP also supports family and consumer groups in building statewide organizations; strengthening their advocacy, mutual support, and education functions; and learning the system well enough to make it responsive to their needs.

In addition to the consumer activities carried out under the auspices of state and national governments, a large network surrounds, supports, and emanates from the mental health consumer movement. It includes the National Mental Health Consumer Self-Help Clearinghouse, based in Philadelphia, which is a resource for self-help groups with support from local agencies and the Community Support Program. In 1993, the CSP also funded a second self-help technical assistance center, the National Empowerment Center, based near Boston. Like the other clearinghouse, it is accessible nationwide through a toll-free telephone number. These nerve centers help link mental health consumers, groups, and resources around the country and provide technical assistance as needed and as resources permit.

Mental health consumers also take advantage of the networking and communication afforded through the telephone, print materials, and conferences. Leaders in the ex-patient movement participate in a CSP-funded monthly teleconference to exchange information and ideas. An Alternatives Conference is held every two years, attended by hundreds of mental health consumers from around the nation. Consumers also participate in Learning Community conferences sponsored periodically by the CSP.

Emerick describes the goals of the most radical (antipsychiatry) faction of mental health self-help as follows: "to change the mental health system away from its traditional individualistic and biological models, toward social and political ones; to politicize the consciousness of former mental patients; and to promote empowered, positive, and non-psychiatric identities through self-help group activities—[including] shedding the sticky 'ex-deviant' labels" (Emerick, 1991, p. 1122). Many of these goals are shared by virtually all mental health self-helpers.

The Community Support Program describes its target population as "individuals 18 years and older with severe mental illnesses (including, but not limited to, schizophrenia, schizoaffective disorders, mood disorders, and severe personality disorders) that substantially interfere with a person's ability to carry out such primary aspects of daily living as self-care, household management, interpersonal relationships, and work or school" (*Harvard*, 1992, p. 3). Consumer-run services, which are partly supported by the CSP, focus on the same population but generally have a broader constituency because drop-in centers, the primary vehicle for consumer services, serve whoever comes for help. The clients and participants of these programs are individuals who might be candidates for hospitalization but are living either at home or in independent living arrangements. Some are homeless.

Former mental health clients Su Budd and Howie the Harp, longtime consumer activists who now coordinate consumer-operated agencies, tell the story of consumer-run programs in an article in *Self-Helper* (Budd and Harp, 1991), published by the California Network of Self-Help Centers. They describe a growing need for specialized help to augment the mutual aid available through self-help groups as poverty and homelessness became more prevalent in the 1980s. Longtime self-help members began to experience burnout, and "many felt that the only way to effectively meet the increased needs was to pay members to provide help."

In addition, "clients . . . found that they liked being with one another" and "began to feel a profound need for a place where they could benefit from peer support every day, not just once a week—a place they could call their own. . . . They also needed funds to pay people and get larger spaces" (Budd and Harp, 1991, p. 2). These conditions led to the creation of drop-in centers, with support from the Community Support Program and state agencies. Some consumer-run programs today have full agency status.

A review of the CSP literature on such programs reveals that a common goal is community integration and improved quality of life and self-esteem for clients with serious mental illness. A common approach is for a state or local agency to use a consumer organization as the contractor for services, thereby enhancing consumer participation in the recovery process. Consumers are used as peer specialists—a vocational category that has been so successful in New York State that it is being added to New York's civil service.

CSP demonstration projects have as a core hypothesis that the participation of consumers is decisive in getting better outcomes. One project abstract states: "The major hypothesis to be tested is that a consumer case management team, because it has had direct life experience interacting with the mental health system, will be as effective as a non-consumer team approach in reducing behavioral symptomatology and in improving a variety of clinical and social outcomes and quality of life for persons served" (Consumer Case Management Demonstration Project, Pennsylvania Department of Public Welfare Office of Mental Health). The outcomes to be studied include social functioning, length and number of hospitalizations, nature and length of employment, nature and number of arrests and convictions, nature of living arrangements, and degree of satisfaction with treatment. This demonstration project is also looking at the secondary impact on consumer case managers, in respect to their job tenure and satisfaction and self-esteem.

The *Harvard Mental Health Letter* interviewed Miles F. Shore, M.D., of the Harvard Medical School and Boston's Massachusetts Mental Health Center for a 1992 report on consumer-operated mental health services. Shore cited the activities of Project SHARE in Philadelphia, On Our Own in Baltimore, the Oakland Independent Support Center, and Denver's Consumer Case Management Program. Their activities and services include case management for former patients, information and referrals to community services, outreach to patients at private psychiatric hospitals, drop-in centers with food and socializing, newsletters, resource libraries, referrals to emergency shelters, independent living support, substance abuse programs, employment counseling, vocational training and placement, live-in residential care, and helpful relationships.

Shore notes that earlier questions about the quality of consumer-run programs have been answered by studies that confirm their effectiveness in increasing work productivity and lengthening the time between hospitalizations.

The shift "from the back wards to the boardroom" (Glover and Steber, 1989) brought about by consumer empowerment can open up new roles and result in tensions in relationships with the people in traditional positions of authority, including professionals, policymakers, and family members. We will examine the implications of consumer empowerment for the mental health system.

Relationships with the Mental Health System

Several areas of interaction with the nation's institutions—policy-making, funding, research, service delivery, and others—are evolving in the self-help arena. Mental health consumers are promoting a variety of changes that affect the services provided, the nature of the provider, research priorities, and financing. They are also demanding changes in the social conditions and attitudes with which they deal, including the elimination of stigmas and discrimination.

Self-help groups' agendas for change are partly a function of their conception of themselves in respect to the mental health system. Some groups see themselves as adjuncts to it, some as partners, some as preferable alternatives, and some as repairers of the damage done by it. Whatever their preferred role, however, the majority of mental health self-help groups are involved in advocacy to bring about specific goals—the closing of state hospitals, control of pharmaceutical prices, antidiscrimination legislation, or public education about a particular disorder.

Directly or indirectly, all are concerned with changing the individual's relationship to a condition and the label attached to it. Among mental health consumers, attitudes toward those labels vary greatly, along with notions of the empowerment they confer. Some groups define their constituencies in terms of medical labels and work to empower members with respect to those conditions. For example, the National Depressive and Manic Depressive Association, as its name implies, serves people with specific diagnoses. Its leaders argue that receiving a correct diagnosis and treatment based on the medical model can be liberating, making possible a return to normal life.

In contrast, members of the ex-patient and survivor movement, while accepting that medication may be necessary, insist that relating to people on the basis of diagnostic labels is more harmful than useful in that it dehumanizes and detracts from more important issues.

Naturally, these and other philosophical differences lead to divergent views about service delivery. The differences apply to both the type of assistance needed and who should provide it. Some ex-patient groups want to be the delivery system for psychosocial services, and in many areas they are doing just that. Other organizations (such as NAMI, the NDMDA, and the ADAA) see self-help as an adjunct to professional treatment and concentrate their advocacy efforts on enhancing and expanding professionally provided services and increasing third-party reimbursement.

Many self-help proponents seek a role for consumers in professionally run service-setting functions such as planning and evaluation. Some go further and want to see an entirely separate system, run exclusively by consumers. Some of these differences get down to the perennial question of whether the system can be reformed from within. For example, the NDMDA has chosen to work with and even within the system. Its leaders cite the organization's impact on pharmaceutical research protocols and the lobbying priorities of the American Psychiatric Association.

Although not all mental health consumers feel equally strongly about consumer-run services, these programs may still be regarded as a touchstone for the system as a whole. How are they different from traditional professional services? A number of ways have been suggested by ex-patient activist Howie the Harp:

> Everyone is equal in power; clients control their individual services, and nothing is done against their will. Clients control the agency in which services are provided; the consumers providing services are role models who understand what clients are going through; clients are recognized as the "real" experts. People are treated with dignity, respect, and fairness: there is tolerance and patience for different types of behavior, including "difficult people"; people are not dealt with clinically or in terms of a diagnosis. Services deal with practical needs and provide practical support; the goal is not cure or

adjustment but improving the quality of the individual's
life [personal interview].

Whatever else it has accomplished, consumer empowerment has
helped abolish the strict dichotomy between professional and
layperson. Today the domain once occupied exclusively by professionals is shared by a multidisciplinary assortment of trained practitioners; "paraprofessionals" with, in some cases, little or no formal
training; and consumers running services.

The taproot of consumer empowerment is its validation of experiential knowledge and the expertise born of "being there" (Borkman, 1976). What role does this leave for the mental health
professional? In answering this question, we must look separately at
two arenas: treatment and governance.

For medical treatment, most self-helpers would encourage their
peers to consult physicians for medical needs, just as one would consult a lawyer or an accountant for other specialized needs. For psychosocial aspects, self-helpers differ as to the proper role of
professionals. Some would not object to consulting professionals,
whereas advocates of consumer-run services stress the importance
of peer support and modeling.

Such differences among mental health consumers, however, are
left behind when it comes to governance and decision making,
where virtually all self-help groups in the mental health arena place
high value on self-determination. There is wide agreement among
self-helpers that professionals cannot control self-help activities.
Self-helpers expect to control governing bodies and budgets and to
participate in all decisions that affect them.

From the professional's perspective, a proper understanding of
roles depends on keeping in mind the diversity of self-help activities and objectives. The relationship between professionals and self-
helpers has many facets. As we noted, consumers are appropriately
autonomous, or at least full partners, in the areas of governance and
advocacy. Professionals are often welcome resources in self-help edu-

cational activities, both for self-education and for outreach to the public. Consultation and referrals are the primary forms of relationship between professionals and self-help groups.

Individually oriented activities such as emotional and practical support and empowerment can be a lightning rod for professional mistrust or competition because to a degree they parallel, augment, or substitute for professional services. Even here, Jacqueline Parrish of the NIMH Community Support Program points out that consumer-run programs are complementary to the formal system, and many people use both (personal interview).

Sometimes mental health professionals are the target of consumer advocacy activity, especially if they are affiliated with mental health institutions or policymaking bodies. In other cases, however, they are implicit or explicit allies in advocacy efforts. There has been much evidence in recent years that professionals have discovered the power of grassroots advocacy and learned to collaborate with consumer groups to press for government funding for research (for example, on schizophrenia) and programs.

In general, the attitude toward self-help among professionals seems to be increasingly receptive, albeit with areas of concern and disagreement. And even the natural tensions between professionals and consumers constitute a healthy dialectical relationship that is one of the creative forces emanating from the self-help movement. This dynamic of two-way learning should be encouraged, not suppressed or smoothed over.

Alfred Katz discusses what professionals have to learn and speculates on the reasons for their resistance. He observes that "professional care systems have tended to monopolize definitions, diagnoses, and treatment of the problems people face. Because of this tendency professionals have deemphasized their clients' self-understanding, self-management, and self-reliance and have thus fostered dependency and passivity. Some professional programs have been notably ineffective. . . . Professionals have also tended to downplay or overlook the need for community, which involves identification and interaction with a like-minded population" (Katz, 1993, p. 71).

Katz later turns from philosophical differences to more material sources of resistance—stating, for example, "It is apparent that these criticisms stem from the groups' challenge to the monopolistic position and self-perceptions of professionals and established institutions in the community" (Katz, 1993, p. 76). He challenges professionals to recognize that "what self-help groups do for their participants . . . is different in kind from what occurs in contacts with professionals and institutions. The self-help experience is unique, a fact that all people concerned with human-services programs must recognize and appreciate" (Katz, 1993, pp. 77–78).

The *Harvard Mental Health Letter* points out that although some professionals perceive, with some justification, a history of mistrust and even conflict between professionals and consumers, "cooperation has been a more constant theme. In general, members of self-help groups use more instead of fewer professional services than other people do, and since the 1970s cooperation has become close. A third of existing groups began with the help of a professional" (*Harvard*, 1993, p. 2).

The article outlines the benefits of cooperation to providers, both individual and institutional—including improved community relations, learning where their services have been inadequate, publicity and referrals, support for patients that augments professional services, and a source of discharge support.

The same article points out the critical role of self-help clearinghouses in creating a bridge between consumers and professionals. From that vantage point, Edward Madara, director of the American Self-Help Clearinghouse, speaks with authority about the importance that professionals, if they are to "form partnerships without compromising the essential nature of self-help," understand "the underlying principles of self-determination and empowerment that contribute to the very life and success of these groups" (interview by author).

Glover and Steber (1989) stress that to accomplish this, the mental health system must move beyond token representation of consumers on advisory and planning boards. Consumers, they say, must be prepared and supported to participate fully and must be given an equal share in decision making. At the heart are issues of control—the issue of "who speaks for the primary consumer." The same authors note that the increasing demand for consumer-operated services is intensifying the competition with professionals for mental health funding for services. It is worth noting that here is where health care reform, which seems to be cleaving closely to the medical model, may set back the flourishing of consumer-run services.

Prevention

One of the major functions of self-help groups is prevention. At the simplest level, all involvement in self-help groups acts to prevent further dysfunction, and in some cases, such as the control of alcoholism, the potential impact is significant in saving lives, reducing accidents, and curtailing serious illness. In general, it should be noted, however, that the preventive focus of self-help typically begins with dealing with a problem or concern, be it the pain of widowhood or the disruption of alcoholism. This is unlike the prevention movement, in which the promotion of wellness does not necessarily begin from an existing malady.

The overall role of self-help in relation to prevention is best seen in the prevention equation adapted from George Albee (1981):

$$\frac{\text{Incidence of}}{\text{dysfunction}} = \frac{stress + constitutional\ vulnerabilities}{\text{social supports} + \text{coping skills} + \text{competence}}$$

The equation suggests two major strategies for preventing dysfunction: decreasing stress or constitutional vulnerability (or both) and increasing social supports, coping skills, and competence (Swift, 1979). Self-help groups provide social support to their members through the creation of a caring community, and they increase members' coping skills through the provision of information and the sharing of experiences and solutions to problems.

This accents what can be done with regard to the denominator of the equation, by strengthening social supports, coping skills, and competence. Prevention theorists sometimes overlook what might be done in relation to the numerator, or at least the stressor portion of it. In many cases, of course, stressors cannot be eliminated or reduced: illness or death of a loved one, accidents, and economic setbacks are not easily controllable. But here we must consider the empowering attributes of self-help groups and their advocacy orientation. This allows for the possibility that the groups may strive for institutional and social changes, which may, in fact, affect stressors such as accidents and economic events such as unemployment.

For example, the self-help group Mothers Against Drunk Drivers (MADD) is concerned not simply with mutual support of people who have lost children to drunk drivers; it is also concerned with making an impact on legislation and other forms of institutional change. So, too, Parents of Murdered Children of New York State is concerned with affecting legislation in that state including a victims' bill of rights. In the home of the woman who started the program, Odile Stern, a bumper sticker on the wall says it all: "Stop the American Handgun War" (*New York Times*, June 4, 1984, p. 17).

Self-help groups exist in a variety of areas that have clear implications for prevention: there are groups for the unemployed, for the parents of premature children, for the families of the mentally ill, for the divorced, for single parent, for smokers or overeaters who want to give up their habit, and for high school and college students, to mention but a few.

Groups for New Mothers

A study of the effectiveness of mutual aid in helping new mothers improve their coping skills sheds important light on the preventive implications of the self-help model (Gordon and others, 1965). A total of 298 mothers who belonged to mutual-support education groups experienced less emotional distress in the six months after childbirth than 362 control subjects did, and their infants were healthier (Parkes, 1972). Follow up studies four to six years later showed that compared with the control subjects, the new mothers in the experimental self-help groups had maintained their emotional gains, had subsequently given birth to greater numbers of healthier children, and had suffered fewer physical illnesses, marital conflicts, sexual problems, and divorces. The data showed that although preparing for problems of postpartum adjustment is helpful to new mothers, developing a self-help network is more critical.

Groups for the Widowed

Bereavement following the death of a spouse has been recognized as a period of extreme stress during which the surviving spouse is vulnerable to emotional and physical illness, particularly in the months immediately following the loss. Research shows heightened impairment in widowed persons' mental health (Parkes, 1964; Clayton, 1974; Cary, 1977; Van Rooijen, 1981) and physical health (Marris, 1958; Maddison and Viola, 1964) when compared to married populations of the same age.

In the past fifteen or so years, a growing number of self-help groups have been established to serve the needs of the widowed, including NAIM (a Catholic-sponsored organization), THEOS (They Help Each Other Spiritually), Widowed Persons Service, Widow-to-Widow, and Community Centers for the Widowed.

Lieberman and Borman (1991) report that active participation in THEOS positively affects the mental health status of the members. Both current and former THEOS members who helped each other through their social network consistently showed better outcomes on seven variables: depression, anxiety, somatic symptoms, use of psychotropic drugs, self-esteem, coping, and mastery. Similar findings were demonstrated in a two-year study of postbereavement adaptation by 162 widows (Vachon and others, 1980).

The importance of these findings is underscored by the size of the population currently and potentially at risk. The twelve million widowed persons in the United States already amount to almost 5 percent of the total population. The projected increase in the size of the older population suggests that the proportion of widowed persons will continue to increase.

The foregoing studies have dealt with acute mental health needs; the following project demonstrates a self-help approach to a chronic condition. With the growth of deinstitutionalization, self-help groups are bridging the gap between hospitalization and community living for ex-patients.

The Community Network Development Project at the Florida Mental Health Institute illustrates how creation of a mutual aid network can reduce hospital recidivism among mental health clients (Gordon and others, 1982). The project's development was guided by the belief that a self-help program for aftercare clients should strengthen the members' abilities to take an active part not only in their own rehabilitation but also in the rehabilitation of their peers.

The project consisted of the establishment of a mutual aid network of self-help groups for aftercare clients. Members of the support groups were trained in leadership and given responsibilities such as teaching psychoeducational classes, telephoning members to remind them of the next group meeting, driving members to meetings, baking cakes for the group, and arranging outings. Not only did this program help individuals improve their personal functioning, but it also contributed to the survival of the group.

Eighty patients who were being discharged from a nine-week intensive treatment unit were randomly assigned to the project or to a control group for traditional aftercare services. Both groups received equivalent discharge planning, including appropriate referrals to a local mental health center for follow-up treatment, if necessary. The groups did not differ significantly according to age, sex, race, marital status, diagnosis, previous hospitalization, or length of follow-up time. At an average follow-up interval of ten months, only one-half as many project members as control subjects had required rehospitalization (17.5 percent versus 35 percent), and their average length of stay was less than one-third as long as that of the controls (7 days versus 24.6 days). Finally, twice as many project members were able to function without any contact with a mental health system (52.5 percent versus 26 percent).

Research Issues

Perhaps the most significant thing to say about self-help research is that in keeping with self-help principles, consumers are taking an increasing part in selecting the questions to be studied and conducting the research. This is particularly true of mental health consumers and ex-patients, some of whom are active researchers.

For consumers, the two chief reasons for conducting research are to identify the conditions under which self-help is most effective and to gain legitimacy for self-help in the eyes of the people who control resources. Human services professionals and policymakers may also wish to determine whether self-help is in fact effective, but consumers accept the answer as self-evident. Another set of questions that may be of interest to all constituencies concerns the cost effectiveness of self-help.

Self-help groups do cost less. In a survey of mental health drop-in centers, social support services provided at consumer, peer-run centers cost approximately $250 per person per year, exactly half the cost in similar professionally run centers (Kaufman, 1993).

The incidence of premature or unnecessary institutionalization of elders may be reduced in families participating in self-help groups. There are potential economic benefits to the community by strengthening the capabilities of home-caregiving families. If each new self-help group delayed the nursing home placement of only one elder for only one year, this would save the $15,000 estimated annual cost of such care. Considering that 38 percent of Americans aged sixty-five and older rely solely on public coverage of personal health-care costs and an additional 60 percent rely on a combination of public and private funding, any reduction in institutionalization of the elderly would save taxpayers a substantial amount.

Lieberman (1986), among others, has explored the difficulty of conducting scientifically valid studies of self-help groups. These research issues, which are discussed at some length by Powell (1993), stem from the fluid and voluntary nature of self-help groups. The *Harvard Mental Health Letter* describes several instances of "unsystematic research" and concludes that "scientific research on self-help groups is largely useless or impossible" because groups are heterogeneous [and] changeable, do not keep records, and have no distinct starting or ending point (*Harvard*, 1993, p. 2).

Both the methodological challenges posed by these factors and the philosophical ones posed by self-helpers' insistence on benefiting from and participating in research make it essential that new research paradigms continue to evolve. The findings of recent collaborative research funded by the Services Research Branch of the National Institute of Mental Health should contribute to this evolution and provide useful information. These projects apply a new research paradigm, in which consumers—also the subjects, generically speaking—select the questions to be studied, are involved in conducting the research, and serve on advisory boards. Knowledge dissemination is also built into the project design so that self-helpers as well as other parts of the mental health system can derive maximum benefit from the findings.

Although they have employed varying methodologies, a number of studies over the past decade have confirmed the efficacy of self-help groups (Kurtz, 1990; Medvene, 1990). The groups studied include THEOS, for widows; caregivers to frail elderly parents; GROW and the National Alliance for the Mentally Ill, for mental patients; and Recovery, Inc. Documented positive outcomes of self-help group participation are in the areas of improvement of functioning, coping, life satisfaction, and stress reduction; amelioration of symptoms; reduction of treatment service use, including hospitalization; assistance for families in positive self-image, building supportive bonds, and coping; improved abstinence and reduction in problem behavior; and increased social networks and employment rates.

One important finding of earlier research is that the individuals who benefit most from self-help group participation are those who participate most actively and are most committed (Rappaport and others, 1985; Videcka-Sherman and Leiberman, 1985; Galanter, 1988). The implicit variation in the quality of participation is important to bear in mind when questions of efficacy are considered.

Even if the scientific evidence in self-help efficacy is still limited, the human services system in recent years has given several expressions of confidence that self-help is an appropriate and effective intervention. An early vote of confidence, as well as a boost to the growing self-help movement, came from Dr. C. Everett Koop when he was surgeon general of the United States. In 1987, Koop invited 175 self-help activists, scholars, and facilitators to a national workshop on self-help and public health. Demonstrating a vision that is not yet realized, he predicted that self-help would come to play a partnership role with health care institutions in promoting public health. "I think that eventually self-help will be the 'other' health system in this country and that it will accept the burden of disease prevention and health promotion in the United States" (*Social Policy*, 1987).

Jacqueline Parrish points out that "even without definitive research on the effectiveness of self-help, health care organizations, state governments, and foundations (Robert Wood Johnson awarded a major replication grant to GROW [in 1989]) are beginning to provide financial and other support to self-help groups" (interview by author). Included in this support is that provided by the National Institute of Mental Health itself.

Parrish adds that "since 1982, the Michigan Department of Mental Health has supported twenty-five consumer-run demonstration projects; twenty-three are still operating. Findings have shown that consumers can successfully operate a wide variety of programs that meet many of their important unmet needs. Their productivity was judged to be high and the cost of the services very low."

In addition—thanks in part to advocacy by the National Council on Self-Help and Public Health (an outgrowth of the surgeon general's workshop)—the federal government's Healthy People 2000 Objectives, developed in the late 1980s through a consensus process, include three for self-help (objective 17.14, regarding self-help opportunities for people with diabetes and chronically disabling conditions, and objectives 6.6 and 6.12, which call for access to self-help groups and statewide clearinghouses for people with mental disorders).

We have already noted that government support for the activities of NIMH's Community Support Program has been sustained for over a decade, bolstered by advocacy by the National Alliance for the Mentally Ill and other groups (Katz, 1993, p. 47). Currently, the CSP funds grants to two technical assistance centers for self-help for mental health consumers, in addition to providing funds for consumer-run programs in every state in the country.

We will conclude our discussion of research by returning to a recurring theme: the evolving role of consumers. Caroline Kaufman urges that consumer review and approval become integral parts of the development and evaluation of human subject issues in clinical services research (Kaufman, 1993). She notes that consumer involvement in the design, implementation, and dissemination of research leads to the need to renegotiate the rights and duties of investigators and consumers. Consumers are no longer merely the objects of research. Although research subjects now have codified rights, "requirements for informed consent have limited application to the more involved roles developing out of recent experiences with participatory research strategies, particularly in the area of self-help group research. The new roles emerging from the consumer advocacy and community mental health movements develop out of shifts in power made concrete by changes in priorities for funding research. . . . This movement goes beyond informed consent and the protection of human subjects to the incorporation of consumer experiential knowledge as a basis for inquiry and understanding of mental illness and its treatment" (Kaufman, 1993, p. 29).

Discussion

At this stage of development, the challenge for self-helpers as well as students and proponents of self-help is to recognize and promote its embeddedness in our social institutions while preserving its distinct, noninstitutional character. Although this is the case for all forms of self-help, the issues are clearly drawn in the mental health context because of consumers' extensive involvement in the related activities of research, service delivery, administration, and policy development.

Virtually every component of self-help has a dimension through which it draws on and collaborates with external resources. Individual support activities have a natural link to professional treatment. Advocacy for patients' rights is institutionalized in protection and advocacy programs. A network of clearinghouses, publishing ventures, and media relations supports and overlaps with the public education and outreach functions of self-help. And consumer advocacy activities are linked to a host of political efforts around housing, health care, criminal justice, and other concerns. Even a superficial review of these connections reveals the embeddedness of self-help in American life.

Yet herein lies the challenge, if not the threat, to the self-help ethos. Although the very term *self-help* is, as explained at the outset, variously applied (contributing greatly to the difficulty of conducting meaningful research), agreement might be reached on the core principles of self-determination, shared leadership, and the minimal exchange of money for self-help services. These principles are at risk in the extensions of self-help into institutional forms and activities.

The challenges of preserving self-help integrity are addressed by Su Budd and Howie the Harp in their 1991 *Self-Helper* article. After describing the growth of self-help agencies from "peer-run and advocacy-oriented" roots, they ask whether today's programs have "stayed true to their roots as they became part of a system they once rejected." The authors offer consumer-run programs a number of suggestions for staying true to their roots: they can "make clear to funders what they will and will not do"—for example, client-run programs do not use or report diagnoses, and no part of the program is compulsory; "adopt innovative structures which express their uniqueness"; and "reflect self-help principles in all aspects of their staffing, management and administration"—for example, with client-controlled boards (Budd and Harp, 1991, p. 4).

However, these goals can be achieved only if self-help principles are clearly and consistently articulated. And even if this happens, it is an open question whether such principles can prevail in the complex environment of an agency. A related set of issues stems from the "commodification" of services in consumer-run programs. Though subsidized services are not commodities to their users, the consumers who provide them are paid. A commitment to consumer empowerment and shared leadership, not to mention a willingness to challenge public policy, may be difficult to sustain when one's financial stability depends on running programs. Placing self-helpers in staff positions also contributes to the entrenchment of certain individuals and militates against shared leadership and mutual accountability—two other important self-help principles.

We are not suggesting that the successes described throughout this chapter as consumers have moved into positions of authority and leadership in the mental health system are not to be celebrated. We are merely asking, Will success spoil self-help?—or more accurately, How can that outcome be avoided? Becoming institutionalized and gaining access to resources are natural and appropriate forms of success for grassroots groups, ones that will enhance the human services sector. But some forms of evolution may be seen in tension with, or even outside the scope of, self-help principles. Clearly, the extensions mentioned here can necessitate a stretching of some core self-help principles. Sometimes success will relegate consumer-operated programs to a hybrid status somewhere between mutual aid organization and public institution or agency. In these cases, an especially close eye must be kept on the type of leadership being provided and the extent to which members share in problem solving and decision making.

Conclusion

There are two outstanding developments in the self-help arena of mental health: the pronounced advocacy that has marked this field and the fact that perhaps the most stigmatized group, mental health patients, has been in the forefront of developing a new form of service whereby mental health consumers provide help to clients and frequently manage their own programs while doing so.

6

Toward a New Education Paradigm

That schools are in a long-term crisis is the ultimate truism, repeated ad nauseam for thirty years. Head Start does not have enough teachers; classes are too large; high school graduates cannot write a decent letter or comprehend an essay written at the level of the *New York Times*.

It is apparent that the schools need more help—resources, money, staff, knowledge. However, over the past two decades, with increased funding, schools have not done a significantly better job. This may be due to the new tasks the schools are required to deal with, such as combating teenage pregnancy and providing AIDS education. But in an era of limits, with enormous attention focused on reducing the federal budget deficit, the chances for large increases in funding for the schools do not seem to be imminent.

Perhaps we have been approaching the problem from the wrong end. Perhaps the question is not What can be done to help our schools? but rather What unused resources already exist in the educational system that will help the schools help themselves?

We would suggest, therefore, that instead of putting all our hopes and energies onto the funding bandwagon, we give serious thought to a powerful educational resource that is ready for the

---

This chapter was written with Audrey Gartner.

taking—one that will go a long way toward helping reduce our nation's educational deficit. This resource exists within the very woof and warp of the school system; it is the students themselves.

What we are suggesting, in brief, is an *institutional self-help model* based on cross-age tutoring: older kids teaching younger kids.

Peer tutoring has been a common practice in Western schools for many years, and it nicely fits our criterion of a self-generated educational resource. Witness the one-room schoolhouse in early America or the modern Montessori method in which children in the higher grades are specially prepared to tutor lower-grade schoolmates.

An example of the basic method of peer tutoring was pioneered during the early nineteenth century, first in England and then in the United States, by the Quaker educator Joseph Lancaster. Central to his approach was the training of senior pupils to instruct younger students using what Lancaster called the monitorial system. A single fully trained child "monitor," Lancaster claimed, could teach one thousand pupils the three *R*'s at a cost of only seven shillings per pupil. (Even in those days, cost effectiveness in the classroom was a virtue not to be ignored.)

More recently, Henry Levin and his associates at Stanford University found that traditional peer tutoring was significantly more cost-effective than computer-assisted learning, smaller classes, and lengthened school time (Levin, Glass, and Weister, 1984). The simple reason was that both tutees and tutors improved their achievement scores for the same dollar input.

A simple but effective technique, peer tutoring brings individualized instruction to the crowded classroom environment, increases time on task, and uses the students themselves to facilitate their own learning. By so doing, it puts unused resources to work and thus addresses one of the basic problems of our time: need and demand are outdistancing availability among human service personnel.

The usual approach to this dilemma is to bring in more technology to expand these resources or to make its delivery more efficient, less wasteful, and less bureaucratic. Here, however, we are witnessing an entirely different approach whereby the release, development, facilitation, and organization of hitherto free resources are put to use from—and in—the very environment that needs this help.

This recycling of latent assets within the structure itself can be seen as the essence of the self-help process. What is changed is not only the quantity of the resource pool but its quality as well—in this instance, the education a child undergoes and, as we shall see, the quality of the school ethos that surrounds it.

Now, if not exactly a fixture in our contemporary school system, peer tutoring has gained a modest, though generally positive, reputation among educators. This is interesting in light of the fact that the influence of child-on-child interaction has been given such short shrift when compared with the parent-child relationship. According to Roger and David Johnson, "Child-child relationships have been assumed to be, at best, relatively unimportant and, at worst, unhealthy influences" (Johnson and Johnson, 1983, p. 123).

In many cases, the influence of peer interactivity has not just been ignored but has been branded as unwholesome and even dangerous. "Not only has this negative bias toward peer influence been reflected in the ways our schools are structured to encourage an adult-child dyadic teaching situation," writes Bonnie Benard, "and to discourage (and even punish) student-to-student interaction, but certainly in the substance abuse prevention field peer pressure has often been viewed as an evil compared to 'Just say no,' rather than as an acknowledgment that peer influence can be a powerful positive force" (Benard, 1990, p. 2).

Criticism and neglect notwithstanding, a growing mass of research data suggests that peer interaction is far more important developmentally than has previously been suspected, "conducive, perhaps even essential, to a host of important early achievements" (Damon and Phelps, 1989, p. 73). Positive peer interactions help establish useful social skills, develop individuation and autonomy, teach youngsters the arts of caring and service, and may help mold a child's sense of right and wrong. According to Johnson and Johnson, "The primary relationships in which development and socialization take place may be with peers" (Johnson and Johnson, 1983, p. 126).

We know from a number of studies that young people generally prefer the help of peers to pedagogical or parental authority figures. For example, a 1986 study of six hundred teenagers at the Emory University Medical Center in Atlanta showed that 70 percent of teens would rather talk with people their own age than with adults. In the same survey, parents were asked whom their children preferred to confide in. Fifty percent of the questioned mothers and fathers chose themselves—but only 20 percent of their children agreed. The rest said that they would rather share their intimate thoughts with friends. Why would a young person threatened with a pressing life problem prefer to listen to the advice of a callow sixteen-year-old contemporary than to that offered by a qualified adult or a loving parent?

The reasons are the perennial classic ones. For much of the past century, American parents have been banished to the outer orbits of their children's social solar system, strangers in a hostile galaxy where differences in language, music, hairstyles, clothes, entertainment, mating habits, and worldview keep the generations apart. Exhorted from an early age to become independent, assured by teen-oriented songs and films that young people really know the truth whereas grown-ups are foolish despots whose primary intent is to persecute youth and blow up the world, such concerns as privacy, autonomy, and peer support ultimately become as important to teenagers as food and drink.

To what extent this adversarial posture benefits society is not our present concern. What is interesting to note, however, is that although the generational conflict is basic and painful, a major principle of self-help lies behind it, namely, that human beings are more likely to reveal their inner thoughts and feelings to people who share their own culture than to outsiders. In short, young people prefer the help and guidance of other young people because they belong to the same culture, the same generation, the same tribe.

A New Peer Model: Reciprocal Tutoring

A considerable body of data indicates that peer tutoring is effective and that tutees improve academically and socially (see Bloom, 1984; Cohen and others, 1982; Gartner and Riessman, 1993; Greenwood and others, 1989; Hedin, 1987; and Swengel, 1991). It is ironic that the effectiveness of the approach may be responsible, in part, for its use primarily as a remedial add-on or relatively peripheral activity. It is typically regarded as a "nice" program, while its potential power is totally ignored. The new peer model, reciprocal tutoring, endeavors to demonstrate this tremendous unrealized power and to present concrete steps toward its realization.

First, a bit of history regarding the "old" peer-tutoring model and the reasons for its effectiveness. Peer tutoring increases time on task and uses the similarity of tutee and tutor to full advantage. In most cases, high-achieving students help low achievers. And therein lies one of the difficulties. Many children approach being tutored with trepidation. Will they fail again? Are they simply stupid? This undercurrent reduces their motivation and involvement.

By contrast, the tutor role reinforces status and confidence. And interestingly enough, tutors have been found to gain genuine benefits from playing this role. This was demonstrated most convincingly in an experiment conducted by Robert Cloward in 1963 at Mobilization for Youth, an antipoverty program in New York City. The critical element in this innovative research was the use of underachieving high school students to tutor underachieving elementary school students in reading. The most telling result of this study was the marked improvement of the high school students, who, in a period of less than five months, improved their scores an average of three years; tutees improved approximately six months (Cloward, 1976).

What was going on here? Through the act of teaching, tutors were gaining scholastic acumen; they were learning how to organize their thinking, plan ahead, set priorities, and direct other people in a helpful way. Through teaching, they were learning to learn. By acquiring the confidence and self-esteem that come as a matter of course from success, a group of disenfranchised, underprivileged youngsters became empowered perhaps for the first time in their lives, with correspondingly positive behavior to show for it.

The significant point made by the Cloward study is that tutoring appears to produce a qualitative leap in the tutors' learning. For this to take place, of course, it is necessary that tutors have room to improve, that they do not enter the tutoring relationship at the ceiling level. If most tutors are already high achievers, they can only show improvement in some other category that is unlikely to be measured in most studies. If, conversely, the tutor is an underachiever or an average student, a much greater growth potential exists. As a result of the Cloward experiment and other studies, the Peer Research Laboratory of the Graduate School and University Center of the City University of New York, codirected by Frank Riessman and Audrey Gartner, has developed a new and highly effective educational paradigm.

This new model is designed to give all students the opportunity to be tutors (and thereby benefit from learning through teaching) and to have all tutors experience the tutee role as part of their "apprenticeship" for becoming tutors. The main features of the "old" and "new" models are shown in Table 6.1.

To test whether the tutoring process actually affects the learning of tutees, we conducted an experiment in six New York City high schools under the auspices a citywide dropout prevention program. In three experimental schools, tutees participated in group meetings with their tutors to discuss the tutoring experience and to

Table 6.1. Tutorial Models: The Old Versus the New.

Old	New
1. Tutees make incremental academic progress via a one-on-one "smart kid, dumb kid" tutorial style.	1. Tutors have the opportunity to make a qualitative leap in learning.
2. Tutees learn by receiving.	2. All students have the opportunity to learn through teaching.
3. Tutoring is essentially a peripheral activity and a remedial add-on.	3. The tutoring process is a central educational strategy involving a broad range of students.
4. Tutees experience feelings of dependency and powerlessness within the tutorial environment.	4. Helpees no longer feel inadequate or dependent. The dominant-passive approach is replaced by "I win, you win, we all win."
5. Repeat tutees are often labeled as losers and may become early school dropouts.	5. The tutee role is temporary and is a developmental step in becoming a tutor.
6. The tutoring program has little impact on overall school culture but rather is confined within the classroom setting.	6. Peer tutoring affects the ethos of the school and flows over into the community at large. The stress is now on cooperation, communication, and mutual aid. Competition, fragmentation, and disunity have become outmoded. The system changes from the ground up through its own efforts and resources.

consider their possible future role as tutors. In three control schools, the tutees were part of a traditional tutoring program.

The results were dramatic; the tutees in the experimental schools received significantly higher grades in the tutored courses, passed more courses, and had better attendance. The tutees also demonstrated a better understanding of the course material. As one tutor expressed it: "I thought I was going to teach by telling, but my tutee actually showed an interest in learning by asking questions rather than just trying to get by."

Reciprocal tutoring is being applied in another Peer Research Laboratory project designed for new immigrant students entering New York City high schools. Typically, immigrant students feel estranged because of their unfamiliarity with the norms and unspoken rules of both the culture and the school. Each new student in this study is paired with a trained high school tutor-mentor who serves as a personal guide, "translating" the school culture. For example, mentors explain what is expected of students by teachers and other school staff, as well as how to study for an exam. In their mentor role, they walk their mentees through the system and acquaint them with their community; as tutor, they help tutees with their academic work. In the semester that follows, tutees then have the opportunity to become tutor-mentors for a new group of immigrant students.

Reciprocal tutoring is being implemented and made more accessible to a broad range of students, including those in special education. For example, in an elementary school, whole classes of sixth graders tutor whole classes of fourth graders, who in turn tutor second grade students. As students progress through the grades, they tutor younger students. This across-the-board learning system spreads the tutoring experience and allows the students to be both givers and receivers of help. On the secondary level, the Peer Research Laboratory undertook a project to determine whether there would be differences in effectiveness among tutors from high-, middle-, or low-achieving high schools in a cross-age (elementary through middle school) tutoring program. Results showed no significant differences.

Another approach is intraclass tutoring, where the tutor-tutee roles are alternated on a regular basis to ensure that all students share giving and getting. Half of the students are prepared to tutor the rest of the class one to one in a particular subject area, while students not being trained read a book, work on a class project, or review a particular skill (all preparatory to being a tutor). At another time, tutor and tutee roles are reversed.

The tutoring approach promotes active learning. Tutors need to rework the material and present it in a way that is understandable to others. Reciprocal tutoring is built around this premise. By adding the requirement that all tutors first be tutees, the experiential base for tutor-centered learning and understanding is built in. If tutors are fully engaged in this process, they acquire not only a deepened understanding of the material that they are presenting but also an understanding of learning how to learn.

Tutors need the opportunity to reflect continually on their experiences, sharing their feelings and thoughts about the tutoring process in group discussions and in personal journals, to fine-tune their skills. In this way, tutors gradually become aware of learning strategies, along with the significance of indirect and informal learning, the relationship between cognitive and social development, the importance of individualizing instruction to attune the subject matter to the learner's interests and learning style, and the use of pacing, repetition, and reinforcement.

The tutees' motivation to learn is similarly enhanced through participatory sharing with tutors, and the value of being tutored in preparation for becoming tutors decreases the asymmetry and stigma often associated with receiving help. Being tutored serves more than "learning the lesson."

Though concerned with a qualitative improvement in learning, the new paradigm is also directed toward an extensive change in the school environment by changing the ethos of the school and by giving greater empowerment to the forgotten constituency, the students. No longer are the students simply acted on; they become major actors. As long as peer tutoring remains a "nice" peripheral activity, this cannot happen. The new paradigm makes the tutoring process a central instructional strategy with a contagious message of sharing and cooperation that affects other constituencies as well, especially the teaching staff. Used in this new way, peer intervention has the potential for satisfying both sides of the debate in regard to the measurement of school change—it can and does significantly improve achievement scores on reading and mathematics and simultaneously affects the entire school environment, replacing passive learners with active students.

The democratizing effect of reciprocal tutoring on teachers has been demonstrated in several of our projects. To make reciprocal tutoring work, the support of the teachers is essential, particularly because of the shift in their role to facilitators of learning—training the students, managing the process, developing a working relationship with their teaching partners, and making the logistical arrangements necessary in cross-age tutoring schemes.

We have found that establishing mutual support groups among teachers not only helps break down teacher isolation but also leads to the development of innovative partnerships and cross-fertilization of ideas among teachers involved in similar work. Support group meetings usually take place before or after school in a relaxed atmosphere where the teachers plan tutoring sessions, discuss tutoring techniques, prepare materials, assess how the tutoring is progressing, and share their feelings about the program's impact on their students and themselves.

Toward a Power Model

So far we have described a basic reciprocal tutoring design. Now we turn to a more advanced model, which embeds peer tutoring in a systematic academic high school course, such as psychology or child development, where the course content consists of both the subject matter and the development of tutoring skills through training and a field practicum.

Although similar in some ways to the reciprocal tutoring model, this power model targets as receivers of help special underserved students who are not necessarily being prepared to be future tutors themselves.

This intensive tutoring model is concerned with providing individualized instruction and with supporting the development of social and cognitive skills for groups in critical situations, such as Head Start and the early primary grades. Although many preschoolers are given a substantial learning boost by Head Start, which has, alas, been severely crippled by funding cutbacks, they are often provided with so little educational follow-through when they enter school that the advantages gained from this important program seep away by the time they reach the second or third grade. A low-cost, long-term, high-payback peer tutoring program might take up the slack.

The tutoring is comprehensive and long-term. It is an essential part of the course in which the tutors are enrolled and of the programs of the younger students. Tutoring is intended to have a major impact. The course approach ensures tutors' continued involvement and provides a substantive knowledge base in relation to both the course subject matter and issues related to learning. This may, among other things, provide stimulation or preparation for a teaching career, thus providing a potential influx of dedicated professionals into the schools. At the very least, these students could become "master tutors," and the tutoring that they introduce should demonstrate the potential power of peer intervention.

Once tutoring has been launched, teachers monitor sessions, attend meetings with tutors, and provide resources, suggestions, and encouragement. Teachers wear many hats in the peer-based world: facilitator, cheerleader, counselor, mentor.

The Peer-Centered School

Peer-based programs, beyond tutoring, are currently being instituted in the schools for drug abuse, after-school child care, alcoholism, antiviolence programs, crisis mediation, student discipline, and community service. Findings show that peer mediation is an excellent method for reducing violence, racial conflict, and verbal abuse both in and out of the classroom (Benard, 1990, p. 2).

Peer-centered programs are also being instituted for suicide prevention, loneliness and friendship issues, overcoming cultural barriers, language adjustment, and sexual awareness. There are many possible variations. In one San Francisco project, students are trained to help other students understand AIDS transmission and risk, then supervised as they pass on what they have learned. An important part of the methodology involves small student-facilitated group meetings at which issues such as abstinence and safe sex are discussed.

How effective are peer-based counseling and mentor programs in the community? An analysis of 143 adolescent drug prevention programs found that "peer helper programs are dramatically more effective than all other [antidrug] interventions" (Tobler, 1986, p. 565).

Despite an enormous amount of data in support of peer learning and the great many peer-based programs currently in operation across the country, there are as yet no fully peer-centered schools in the United States.

If one did exist, how might it operate? What would its day-to-day activities include? In what ways would it differ from regular schools? A peer-centered school would be an educational center where the peer paradigm is applied not only to tutoring but also to the social, administrative, and educational structure of the entire institution. Such a school would have some or all the following features.

1. *Mentor assignment.* New students are assigned upper-grade peer helpers who shepherd them through the difficult first days of school and act in an advisory capacity when problems arise. A typical program might recruit and train high school juniors and seniors to act as guides, advisers, and friends for entering students. When these freshmen reach the upper grades, they are mentors for other new students.

2. *Support groups.* Mutual-support self-help groups are encouraged by the school administration and are facilitated by adults or students (or both). Students meet in "rap rooms" to talk about matters that concern them. These groups may include chapters of existing organizations such as Alateen, Students Against Drunk Driving, and Teens Together. Or support groups can be founded by students on an as-needed basis—for example, a branch of Compassionate Students (who have lost a family member) or groups to deal with issues of career choice, parent divorce, health, stress management, sexuality, relationships, eating disorders, immigration, and so forth.

3. *Student advisory committees.* Students serve on a variety of advisory committees where their voices are heard on governing issues such as suspension, admission policy, and discipline and where they deal as well with issues of academics, peer programs, sports, values, and extracurricular activities.

4. *Interclass cooperation.* Cooperative interclass peer support and interchange are instituted. Included are peer-centered activities such as student coaching, tutoring, and mentoring.

5. *Strategic planning programs.* Students are encouraged to write a strategic plan of action designed to improve their school. For example, they might conduct a student survey regarding perceived educational needs, attitudes toward existing school programs, or suggestions for change. Students working in these programs enjoy

greater empowerment as well as a chance to hone their organizational and planning skills.

6. *Student training*. Students who participate in peer-based programs are trained in whatever subjects are appropriate to the program: research methodology, teaching instruction, counseling, self-evaluation techniques, and so forth.

7. *Interschool cooperation*. Students meet with representatives from other peer-based schools to discuss issues of social and academic policy.

8. *Teacher support groups*. Teacher support groups meet regularly to discuss their peer-based projects, provide time for cooperative planning, and stimulate teacher participation.

9. *Community service*. Students contribute a certain number of hours of community service each academic year. The choice of workplace may include day-care centers, senior centers, hospitals, schools, rehabilitation programs, and parks.

10. *Demonstration training*. To encourage the spread of peer activities and to propagate the peer helper philosophy, the peer-centered school serves as a demonstration training base (DTB) that educators, parents, and students visit to observe peer training in action, learn methodology, participate in activities, and receive assistance in learning how to implement such a model in their own school. In this way, the school becomes a living laboratory and prototype for all interested observers.

Conclusion

If so many persuasive reasons exist for installing peer programs in our schools and if evidence bears out their value, why are they not spreading like wildfire?

There are several reasons. For one thing, peer tutoring and other peer-based programs are little known or understood by parents and educators. They are viewed as a small intervention among many, not as a full-blown alternative and constitutive educational method and philosophy.

Some people believe that student tutors will provide substandard help for tutees and will therefore compromise the educational system with misinformation and bogus teaching methods. However, tutors are allowed to teach only after undergoing a rigorous course of training both in their field of study and in tutoring instruction.

Observers in some educational camps fear that our schools will be "overrun" by teenage tutors or will place too much power in the hands of students. We know, however, that one of the essential elements of the tutoring model—its sine qua non, really—is teacher guidance and input. Without this keystone feature, the entire superstructure tumbles.

Some professionals feel that peer programs place too much power in the hands of students, causing teachers to lose control and possibly even placing their jobs in peril. Again, it must be stressed that teachers, not students, run the peer-based program. Teachers design the programs, train the tutors, and monitor, supervise, and chart the course; without their guidance and approval, the train never pulls out of the station.

Student resources can never be a substitute for adult school personnel. They can, however, supplement the work of professionals, lighten their burden, and in the long run make their teaching chores more compelling, more fulfilling, and more fun.

The critical importance of young people having the opportunity to participate in meaningful roles such as helping other youths is a salient factor in preventing social problems, including substance abuse, teen pregnancy, and delinquency. The need exists to expand the opportunity to have all students experience the helping role.

The new tutoring model is a step in this direction. It calls for in-depth preparation and training of peer tutors and their ongoing reflection on the tutoring process; it removes the negativity usually associated with receiving help, for all students participate in giving and receiving help; it makes being a tutee a prerequisite for becoming a tutor; and it leads to the creation of student-centered, peer-focused schools. An ancillary aim is the spread of other peer opportunities: peer mentoring, peer mediation, peer education, peer helping.

Teachers today appear more receptive to peer-based programs and student decision making than in the past. Perhaps the most important first step, then, in helping teachers and administrators think in new ways about school policy is to help them understand that *they themselves* represent an underused source of educational innovation and that without their input, the student empowerment movement cannot work.

7

Restructuring Help

A commonsense view of help regards it as an interaction in which an explicit intention on the part of one party, the help giver, is to aid another party, the help receiver (Fisher, Nadler, and Whitcher-Alagna, 1982). A more recent definition states that help is "an action that has a consequence of providing some benefit to or improving the well-being of another person" (Schroeder and others, 1995, p. 17). The problem with this formulation is that it omits a vast area of help-getting that is the result of giving help. In fact, paradoxically, it appears to be much easier for someone to give help than to receive it, and it is much more helpful to the giver.

We first observed this phenomenon in self-help mutual aid groups, where an essential part of the self-help ethos called for members not only to receive help but also to give it. This ethos is one important way in which mutual aid groups are unique; it distinguishes them from groups where an individual may receive help and then leave the group, much to the chagrin of group leaders. The essence of the self-help group is giving help and benefiting from giving.

The Helper Therapy Principle Revisited

In its simplest form, the helper therapy principle states that people who give help are helped the most. The alcoholic in AA who provides support to another AA member may benefit more than the helpee by virtue of playing the help-giving role. Furthermore, because all members of the group play this role at one time or another, all are benefited by the helping process. In a sense, this is true of all helpers, be they professionals or volunteers, but it may be more sharply true for helpers who have the same problem as the helpee, as is characteristic of mutual aid groups. Although all help givers may be helped themselves in a nonspecific way by playing the helping role (and this is in itself an important matter), people who have a particular problem may be helped in much more specific ways by providing help to others who have the same specific problem, whether they are alcoholics, drug addicts, smokers, underachievers, heart patients, hypertensives, or diabetics.

As Dewar points out, "It feels good to be the helper. It increases our sense of control, of being valued, of being capable. When children play by acting out help relationships, they are [more] apt to seek to play the role of the helper than [the role] of the helped. It feels better. As a person organizes more of his or her identity around their activities and value as a helper, it gets harder to keep him or her from helping. It always seems more predictable that the helpers will benefit from helping rather than the helped" (Dewar, 1976, p. 23).

Man Keung Ho and Judy Norlin used the helper therapy principle in a children's residential center. They observed that "since meaningful living and encounter require the reciprocal processes of giving and receiving, the helper role provides [residents with] . . . the opportunity to reverse their customary role. . . . Unless they are afforded the opportunity to give, further efforts to help them tend to become futile and dehumanizing" (Ho and Norlin, 1974, pp. 112). This concept is operationalized in a pairing system where older residents are assigned as orienters and guides to new residents and as cotherapists in family treatment and aftercare.

Kelly found that the greater the involvement of a person in the helping process, the greater the positive effect on self-concept (Kelly, 1973).

Weiss, in his study of Parents Without Partners (1973), noted that "both men and women sometimes found that contribution to the organization through service in administrative or planning roles supported their own sense of worth. Leaders referred to this phenomenon by saying, 'The more you put into PWP, the more you get out of it.'" Because PWP recognized that "helping" was therapeutic, it maintained many divisions and programs responsible for their own activities: "This administrative fragmentation made it possible for an administrative position to be offered to almost any member who wanted one, if not as a director of a division, then as a program coordinator or other functionary within one" (pp. 323–324). The same principle, of course, is applied in AA, where leadership is widely diffused; many individuals have the opportunity to play various leadership roles.

The helper therapy principle is operative in many areas outside of self-help. In Chapter Six, we noted its significance in relation to the special benefits to the tutor.

The Helper's High

The helper concept has been considerably expanded in recent years, particularly in the work of Allan Luks (1991), who introduced the term *helper's high*.

A national survey conducted by Luks involving 3,300 volunteers from all fields (helpers of AIDS patients, homeless families, shut-ins, crime victims, runaway youths, hospital patients) led to some interesting findings:

- Nearly 95 percent of the volunteers reported that personal helping on a regular basis gives them an immediate pleasurable sensation. This "helper's high" consists of physical and emotional sensations including a sudden warmth, a surge of energy, and a feeling of euphoria immediately after helping.

- Helper's high is often followed by a longer-lasting phase involving feelings of increased self-worth, calm, and relaxation. Nearly 80 percent of respondents reported that the good feelings would return, in diminished intensity, when the helping act was remembered.

- People who experienced this syndrome reported better-perceived health. Nine out of ten said that they were healthier than other people their own age. Other studies indicate that this perception is one of the strongest predictors of future health and longevity.

- Many helpers also reported fewer colds, headaches, and backaches; improved eating and sleeping habits; and even relief from the pain of chronic diseases such as ulcers, asthma, arthritis, and lupus ("Rx: Helping Others," 1993).

In a study of 2,700 residents in Tecumseh, Michigan, for example, men who volunteer for community organizations were two and a half times less likely to die from all causes of disease than their non-involved peers ("Rx: Helping Others," 1993).

Although these studies add an important dimension to our thesis, it should be clear that the referent is to helping behavior on the part of the volunteer and in no way indicates that the receiver is actually helped. Of course, this is true for the mutual aid examples as well. In the tutoring situation, peer tutoring has been demonstrated to provide consistent improvement on the part of the tutee. And evidence is increasing that mutual aid groups are beneficial. This may be due less to the fact that the help is received and more to the fact that it is given with at least minimal acceptance by the receiver (in self-care, the giver and the receiver are one and the same).

Why Does It Work?

Numerous mechanisms have been postulated to explain the potential power of the helper therapy idea. Seeking to describe and explain the helper therapy principle, Skovholt (1974) summarizes the benefits received from helping: "(1) the effective helper often feels an increased level of interpersonal competence as a result of making an impact on another's life; (2) the effective helper often feels a sense of equality in giving and taking between himself or herself and others; (3) the effective helper is often the recipient of valuable personalized learning acquired while working with a helpee; and (4) the effective helper often receives social approval" (p. 58). Skovholt hypothesizes that all four factors, rather than any one, make the helper therapy principle potent.

Skovholt further sees the helper therapy principle as rooted in social exchange theory and the norm of reciprocity, which is a universal norm, according to Gouldner (1960); essentially, it states that people should help but not hurt those who have helped them. As a norm, reciprocity relies on an economic exchange model, so that one is not in debt to another person. Skovholt suggests that in working with drug and alcohol addicts, who typically violate the reciprocity norm by taking more than they give, the helper therapy principle may have special significance. The strict structure of programs such as AA, with the norm of helping others, may have the result that "for the first time in a long time these members feel a sense of reciprocity and, therefore, satisfaction with themselves" (Skovholt, 1974, p. 63).

The mechanisms probably also vary with the setting and the helper's task. Helpers functioning in a therapeutic context, whether as professional therapeutic agents or as nonprofessional "peer therapists," may benefit from the importance and status associated with this role. Because relationships in a self-help setting between helper and helpee are usually between persons of little status discrepancy and do not involve an exchange of money, Skovholt suggests that the exchange theory of Foa and Foa (1971) may apply. This theory points out that a social exchange does not necessarily mean a loss to one of the two parties. "The helper and helpee can . . . give to each other without either person losing" (Skovholt, 1974, p. 61).

Persuading Oneself by Persuading Others

Helpers in the process of persuading helpees have to persuade or reinforce themselves, not in some general way, but specifically concerning the various problems that they share. King and Janis (1956) found that subjects forced to improvise a speech supporting a specific point of view tended to change their opinions in the direction of this view more than subjects who merely read the speech for an equivalent amount of time. The King-Janis study suggests that becoming committed to a position by advocating it ("self-persuasion through persuading others") may be an important dimension associated with the helper role. Pearl and Riessman (1965) note that many helpers (such as homework helpers in school) are "given a stake or concern in a system," and this contributes to their becoming "committed to the task in a way that brings about especially meaningful development of their own abilities" (p. 232). They observe that community ownership of services is far more empowering than simply being served. For example, when tenants in public housing became the resident managers, the crime rate fell and the general maintenance of the project was enormously improved.

The Helping Role

At least three additional mechanisms account for the fact that the person playing the helping role achieves special benefits: (1) the helper is less dependent; (2) in struggling with the problem of another person who has a like problem, the helper has a chance to observe his or her own problem in perspective; and (3) the helper obtains a feeling of social usefulness by playing the helping role.

The helper therapy concept is derived from role theory, according to which a person playing a role tends to carry out the expectations and requirements of that role. In effect, as a helper, the individual displays mastery over the afflicting condition—plays the role of a nonaddict, for example—and thereby acquires the appropriate skills, attitudes, behaviors, and mind-set. Having modeled this role for others, the individual may see himself or herself as behaving in a new way and may adopt the new role as his or her own.

Helpers also receive support from the implicit thesis that "I must be well if I can help others." There is also an explicit reward in helping others, in having an impact on another person's life, in reducing another's suffering. Moreover, the helper role may function as a major distracting source of involvement, diverting helpers from their own problems and a general overconcern with self.

Why is helping others such a gratifying experience? There are a variety of reasons. Helping provides a sense of usefulness and increased social status. People who lend a friendly hand in self-help groups or volunteer work think of themselves as a needed and admired part of the community. Over time, they come to believe that they have something special to give and a unique ability to make a difference: this in turn provides them with a sense of roots, of purpose, of a place in the sun.

Giving aid to others is an empowering activity. It makes benefactors feel potent, competent, worthy, OK—indeed, it provides them with all the positive therapeutic responses that mental health professionals try to engender in their patients. In this era of global anomie, when people perceive themselves as mere numbers on the rolls of the technostate, serving others reconfirms their sense of identity and control. "After all," helpers tell themselves, "I can't be *that* helpless if I can affect another person's life in such a positive way."

The simple act of giving guidance and comfort to other human beings provides helpers with a veritable cornucopia of the psychic benefits that all of us seek—admiration, status, power, competence, companionship, love, and feelings of self-worth. Helping, in this sense, can be seen as a form of psychological self-medication.

Just how do charity, generosity, and compassion benefit us? A number of psychological mechanisms are at work. By helping others, we may relieve our own distress at the sight of pain or misfortune and prevent stressful guilt feelings. Focusing on others relieves the gridlock of our own family, financial, work, or interpersonal hassles. We get a special kind of attention from the people we help. Most of us need to feel that we matter to someone; sincere gratitude can be very nourishing.

Helping can also block pain, due perhaps to distraction, thanks to our limited capacity to pay attention to several things at once. And because we tend to assess our own situation by comparing ourselves to a select group, helping others expands our perspective and enhances our sense of gratitude for what we have. For example, helping someone less capable may enhance our sense of our own skills, competences, and strengths.

The Helpee Perspective

The help paradox calls attention to the fact that benefits to help givers are often greater than those obtained by help receivers.

The helper's benefits are more consistent, less ambiguous, and often accompanied by extra gains. Tutors may not only improve their own reading level, for example, but also boost their self-esteem, hone their social skills, and make progress in learning how to learn. By contrast, tutees may show only small incremental improvement in reading and express some ambivalence about being perceived as low achievers. Moreover, the two roles themselves have intrinsically different properties, the helper being more independent and the helpee more dependent.

Before going further, it may be useful to clarify certain distinctions. A teacher gives help in the form of teaching; a student receives help by going to class; a student is helped if he or she learns. A helpee may seek help and yet not be helped. Thus we are distinguishing among giving help, receiving help, and actually being helped.

In self-help mutual aid, a relevant finding is reported by Linda Roberts (1989) in her study of GROW. She found that "helping others is associated with improvement over time in social adjustment and in higher attendance, while receiving help did not significantly contribute to any of the outcome variables." Pushed to its extreme, this could mean that in mutual aid interactions, the helpee is no more than a foil or a guinea pig because it is the helper who really benefits. Fortunately, in most self-help groups, many individuals have the opportunity to play the role of the helper part of the time. A possible implication is that the groups would benefit if this norm is maximized, as it is in many twelve-step groups and in Parents Without Partners. Moreover, as individuals have the opportunity of playing the helper role, they may be less ambivalent about receiving help.

All of this leads to the question of the relationship of helper benefits to the benefits the helpee receives in the interaction of the two. Do helpers benefit regardless of what happens to helpees? It may seem so in the description of helper benefits that are reported with no information on the receivers.

Does it matter whether these help receivers are really being helped or not? Even in the most abstract, indirect help-giving—say, donating blood—learning that a patient has improved as a result of the transfusion will affect the help giver differently from hearing that the patient has died on the operating table.

In the extreme, one would assume that if the receivers are unhappy with the help they are getting, this might hinder the operation of the helper therapy principle.

We know that helping does not always help the helper. For example, in burnout syndrome, helpers may express frustration and despair with regard to their helpees or to the bureaucratic structures under which they must work.

The overarching implication of these observations on the possible reciprocal effects of helper-helpee interaction is that the helpee cannot be ignored; the assumption cannot be made that helpers automatically benefit from volunteering. If the consequences for the helpee are significant for the helper therapy principle to operate, considerable attention must be given to helpees and the conditions that maximize their receiving help. Here the work of Fisher and colleagues is important as they survey and analyze the data and experiences that affect help-getting (Fisher, Nadler, and Whitcher-Alagna, 1982).

They note that help is often experienced as a mixed blessing and that situational conditions and recipient characteristics affect reactions to help. On the one hand, "help may be threatening in that it implies an inferiority relationship to the donor that conflicts with self-reliance and independence. On the other hand, it may communicate donor caring and provide instrumental benefits, e.g., money, advice." Further, "when individuals do not anticipate being able to restore equity, they refrain from seeking needed help or are slower to ask for it." Moreover, "many kinds of help are potentially freedom-restricting because they are inextricably linked to beliefs about how one should respond to help—don't bite the hand that feeds you, the reciprocity norm, you don't get something for nothing" (Fisher, Nadler, and Whitcher-Alagna, 1982, p. 114).

In this context, based on our work with student peer helpers, we offer some conditions for accepting help:

1. No stigma should be attached to help that is received. Providing help universally—for example, to all students in the school or all sixth graders—would satisfy this condition.

2. If the help received is embedded in training for another role—for example, preparing a tutee to become a tutor— acceptance of the help is much greater.

3. If the help-receiving situation is temporary, it will be received more readily; for example, in intraclass peer tutoring, half the class receives help from the other half on a concept for which the helping half has received specific instruction. The roles are then reversed so that the tutees become tutors on a different concept for which they have received instruction.

4. If the help receiver has direct control or participates significantly with regard to the help, acceptance is likely to be greater.

5. Mentors are well received. This is because they are able to offer help out of experience but without authority or control over the help receiver. Peer mentors for elementary school youngsters can be recruited from the high school population, and high school seniors can be asked to work with incoming students or new immigrants.

Helpers should be aware that in certain situations, helping can hurt. Sometimes helping serves as so-called enabling behavior, whereby, say, an alcoholic's behavior is in fact perpetuated by the reward of tolerance and support from family and friends. Another well-known situation arises when one spouse consciously or unconsciously keeps the other spouse dependent on his or her "help" and thus under his or her thumb—the classic case of codependency.

Tutees may be hurt by help if they feel stigmatized and labeled as deficient because they need help.

Copious literature exists on iatrogenic effects, the contracting of illness as a consequence of a hospital stay. Another by-product is the dependency that may evolve in any help-receiving context.

Helpers can learn to be effective in their role. Currently, community service programs throughout the country and the National Service Program itself are concerned with improving this help-giving behavior that we call *learned helpfulness*. The National Center for Service Learning has been set up at the Graduate School and

University Center of the City University of New York to assist in the training of service helpers in the school and community.

Learned Helpfulness

We have no ultimate answers here, but we do have plenty of helpful advice that we would like to offer to help givers.

1. Examine your motives for becoming involved in a helping situation. They are probably not entirely altruistic, and that is as it should be. You have the right—one could say the obligation—to profit from this exchange. Just beware of a "saint trip," believing that your motives are pristinely free of all selfish concerns; they almost certainly are not. Understand what you hope to achieve through helping and what you want personally from the interaction.

2. Take a hard look at the people you are helping. Do they want your help? Do they need it? Did they ask for it? Do they like the way it is being offered? Do they seem happy with what is being given? Do they feel put down or left out? Do they perceive themselves as underachievers, underprivileged, underclass, homeless?

3. Does the help you are offering allow recipients to become independent or play the role of helper for others in turn? Or does your support keep people in a permanent state of dependency and obligation? Note here that an exemplary check against this tendency comes built into the mutual aid self-help group dynamic, wherein members frequently change roles, one day playing the helper, next the helpee. Experience tells us that this reversibility of roles is a critical safety device in any interactive situation. Once it is instituted, a balance of power is more easily maintained within groups, learning is shared rather than forced on one person by the next, and the destructive dominator-dominated dichotomy is avoided.

4. Is there a distinct difference in social class between you and the help receiver? Does your behavior in any way emphasize or perpetuate this difference? How might you underplay this discrepancy or make it irrelevant?

5. At times the help process carries hidden agendas such as political bias or a form of advocacy. Such latent elements are not necessarily harmful and may even be helpful. But they must be made explicit from the start if a group is to function in an honest and efficient way.

6. It is important for helpers to acknowledge exactly what they are getting from the helping process: power, learning, recognition, the ability to change the system and make a difference.

What do these many suggestions add up to? Three things: (1) cooperation, caring, and giving are vital elements in the helping interchange; (2) for a support relationship to work, both parties must share in the benefits; and, most of all, (3) if we restructure the character of the help dynamic itself so that it becomes mutual aid rather than one-way giving—if we are no longer driven to be one up but rather allow each participant to play the role of helper and helpee in turn—the very nature of the process will automatically improve.

This means that if help recipients are allowed to maintain a sense of dignity and competence, if they have a voice in things and are not simply passive receivers of charity, and if at times they get to sit in the giver's seat and share in its rewards, that will go a long way toward achieving a harmonious give-and-take.

Conclusion

Two strategies emerge in response to the helping paradox that we have outlined. First, we need to restructure help, to universalize the helper role so that everyone has the chance to be a helper with all of its associated benefits (see Chapter Six). The helper therapy principle remains the most powerful source of help for the individual. Second, helpers require helpees; hence, helpers must understand the helpees' situation, its natural limits as well as the results of receiving poor help. The development of the helpee, like the increased effectiveness of the helper, is improved through understanding the helpee role and through playing both roles in the course of development. Because helpees become helpers, understanding their own roles as helpees should help them become better helpers. Mutual aid groups provide an ideal model for the helper-helpee relationship.

Social Change:
The Personal Becomes Political

The relationship of self-help to social change is complex and controversial. Some critics maintain that the self-help approach is essentially concerned with individual, psychological change and not institutional or social change, that in fact it retreats from the big social picture to a smaller canvas where the individual can feel some degree of empowerment—from long-term objectives to living one day at a time.

In this sense, it is regarded as apolitical. The argument goes something like this: People feel that they cannot possibly affect decisions about the economy or world peace, but they can do something about aspects of their personal life, such as smoking, gambling, or overeating. This view that self-help is nonactivist is directed particularly at Alcoholics Anonymous and its twelve-step model because AA as an organization explicitly disavows political action and social activism. As Ruth and Victor Sidel put it: "While self-help groups are an important and encouraging development, they are often more a response to symptoms than to underlying problems. These problems include the unequal and unjust distribution of resources and power within our society [and] the tendency to blame the victim rather than changing the victim's circumstances" (Sidel and Sidel, 1976, p. 67).

Actually, the self-help approach has been integrally involved in social action and has in fact been in the forefront of positive, progressive social change. Moreover, although AA chooses not to engage in political action as an organization, individual members using AA's philosophy have promoted an enormous range of institutional changes, which will be described in detail later in this chapter.

The Personal Is Political

In the 1960s, the notion that the personal is political became the byword of various movements. In a sense, the self-help movement is the present-day embodiment of this concept. This is most evident in two major movements built on a self-help base: the rights of the disabled and the women's movement. The political issues in each of these movements are frequently, if not exclusively, personal. Each movement essentially began with small self-help mutual aid units—the Centers for Independent Living and women's consciousness-raising groups, respectively. In both cases, the internal identity-strengthening dimension of self-help served as a critical first step that enabled the groups to move outward and ultimately to engage in social and political action. In this context, self-help was a means to the groups' ends and was particularly important in the early stages of their development.

In some instances at least, self-help may serve as a transitionary stage in the process of political engagement. In the self-help phase, a group looks inward to develop its resources, methods of coping, and broad identity, mobilizing inner strengths. The group may then move outward, establish an advocacy stance, and demand changes in the external environment (new laws, institutions, services). At this point, the group sustains a dual self-help and advocacy posture, as in the case of Parents of Murdered Children. Certain groups may go beyond the self-help structure and become more fully advocacy oriented—as, for example, groups of people with disabilities, which, though they may still have some self-help mutual aid features, have essentially become legislatively oriented political organizations.

Personal origins also characterize numerous other significant self-help developments. Mothers Against Drunk Drivers (MADD) began following the death of Candy Lightner's daughter under the wheels of a drunken driver. The group has emerged as a forceful lobby for tough legislation and court action regarding drunk driving.

A similar pattern occurred with community action groups. National People's Action began with local concerns about neighborhood housing, but in pursuing them, it spurred national legislation such as the Community Reinvestment Act, which opposed redlining by banks (a method of denying loans to low-income persons).

Thus the criticisms that the self-help movement is too personal and too local and that it diverts attention from social or structural change ignore the fact that individual change, with its potential power for social change, often begins on a small, personal level and expands from there.

Self-Help and Advocacy

Self-help groups of varying types have made dozens of inroads into individual policy areas. Parents on the Move, Inc., is an example of women organizing and agitating on everything from the crack crisis to the need for better housing. Founded by residents of the Brooklyn Arms, the second-largest welfare hotel in New York City, the group describes itself as women "fighting to get back into society" by securing for themselves decent permanent housing, education, and employment.

A wide variety of victims' rights groups, such as the National Victim Center, have emerged. In New York, victims' groups have been instrumental in the passage of legislation restricting the cross-examination of rape victims about their past sexual history, and they are having similar effects elsewhere in the country.

Disease-centered groups, which were traditionally apolitical, have become politicized by events. For example, Parkinson's groups demanded that tissue obtained from aborted fetuses be utilized in federally funded experiments to test the effectiveness of implanting this tissue in the brains of Parkinson's patients.

The National Association of Atomic Veterans (NAAV) brings together thousands of former members of the armed forces who were exposed to radiation during the three decades of U.S. atmospheric and underground nuclear tests. The NAAV has helped atomic victims become aware of and cope with what has happened to them; at the same time, it has been instrumental in pressing the government to deal honestly with the problem, which it tried for years to ignore.

Self-help is more important than ever in the African-American community. Over a decade of retrenchment on the social justice agenda of the 1960s has given blacks good reason to be cynical about government's interest or ability in dealing with the runaway problems of urban neighborhoods. Many leaders in the African-American community have concluded that it is time to stop relying on help from the outside and look instead to self-help.

Today there are large and increasing numbers of self-help mutual aid groups explicitly oriented toward social change, including Self-Help for the Hard of Hearing, the National Alliance of the Mentally Ill, Disabled in Action, SHARE and other breast cancer and mastectomy groups, the Centers for Independent Living, ACT-UP (for people with AIDS), the Gray Panthers, the Older Women's League (OWL), the National Women's Health Network and the National Black Women's Health Project, DES Action, Vietnam Veterans of America, Victims of Incest Can Emerge Survivors (VOICES), Grandparents'-Children's Rights, the Disabled Women's Network (DAWN), Parents of Murdered Children, the Society of Americans for Recovery (SOAR), the National Association of Caregivers, and Yesterday's Children.[1]

A prime example of how self-help led to social action is exemplified in the Association for Retarded Citizens (ARC). Chapters of ARC were started in the early 1950s as parents' self-help groups. Parents got together because they were disturbed by doctors' telling them to institutionalize their children born with Down syndrome, spina bifida, or other handicaps. "It would be better for both you and the child," they were told. At first, the parents shared mutual concerns: Why did this happen to me? This is tearing my family apart; I can't face my neighbors; I feel guilty. Then they started to look at the options for keeping their handicapped children at home. They created and paid for educational programs until the early 1970s, when their lobbying efforts resulted in legislation guaranteeing every child with a handicap a free and appropriate education in the least restrictive environment possible.

While ARC's legislative efforts continue today, local chapters keep up their mutual support functions. Parents will help one another cope with a difficult situation, but the burden they carry has been made less onerous by their social action.

Another illustration of the self-help social change model is found in various victims' rights groups. Families of homicide victims are some of the most vocal activists fighting for a larger role in the criminal justice system. "When your child is murdered, it's a life sentence of grief, anger, and loneliness that you can never escape," says Odile Stern, cofounder of Parents of Murdered Children of New York State, whose daughter was murdered in the early 1980s. "Then you are thrown into a criminal justice system that . . . doesn't make sense, a system that adds to the original victimization" (from speech presented to Parents of Murdered Children of New York State, November 1983).

Victims' rights activists have organized to change the system. In New York, they supported a bill that restricts cross-examination of rape victims about their past sexual history. The new bill, expanding an earlier rape shield law, was passed unanimously by the state legislature. These activists are now lobbying for an amendment to the state constitution that will give victims and

their families more say in the case against their assailant throughout the trial and sentencing.

Currently, women with breast cancer, emulating the militancy
of people with AIDS in ACT-UP, have formed the National Coali-
tion of Cancer Research and are lobbying for more federal and state
attention to their illness. One of their advocacy groups is called Y-
ME. An older mastectomy self-help group called SHARE over a
decade ago fought insurance companies and employers that discriminated against patients who had had a mastectomy.

Neither Left nor Right

Support and criticism of self-help do not divide neatly along conservative, liberal, or radical political lines. The Bush administration
was attracted to self-help as an economical alternative to costly government programs, and as far back as 1980, the Republican party
adopted a plank in its platform calling for more self-help initiatives.
The Republicans, however, have an ambivalent stance toward self-
help, and it is easy to understand their skittishness when we consider that the political slant of many self-help groups is decidedly
progressive.

But liberals are also divided on the self-help movement. Many
traditional liberals are troubled by its antistate bias, the rejection of
experts (who form an important part of the liberal constituency),
and the possibility that self-help may be used as a substitute for
urgently needed services. Self-help's tendency to direct energies
toward reforming the individual rather than society has provided a
further ground for discomfort among liberals.

Some people on both sides of the political aisle have charged
that self-help deals with symptoms rather than causes, concentrating on the small picture but missing the big one. Without a broad
social vision, how can they address, for instance, the way that the
unequal distribution of wealth and services in our country has led
to the deterioration of the cities? Or for that matter, how can peer

groups of people with chronic illnesses truly address the shortcomings of our health care system?

This criticism is of greater concern. Is self-help a detour from dealing with the major problems of society at their source? Perhaps. But it may very well be that in many cases, this detour is only a temporary retreat that comes from feeling that issues like the economy and the environment are too big and unmanageable for the average person to handle. For many people, self-help can be an attempt to reduce the daunting complexity and seriousness of these important issues to a more accessible and human scale. It is a way for something to be done now, through individual initiative. From there, the next evolutionary step is the transfer of those skills and that group energy and imagination to a larger social canvas.

The fact that criticism of self-help comes from all sides is perhaps as much a reason for hope as for concern. Cutting across traditional liberal-conservative orthodoxies, self-help may represent a fresh, independent form of political energy, a new way of addressing old problems. But what is needed is neither trivial acceptance nor simplistic rejection but rather a serious examination of what self-help does and does not do.

The essence of self-help is the emphasis on the potential inner strength of the individual, group, or community. The criticism that the self-help movement is too tightly focused on the personal greatly underestimates the powerful role of individual change in the process of social change.

AA and Institutional Change

AA's staunch refusal to associate itself with causes, ideologies, public policy, publicity, fundraising, business, and the political rough-and-tumble has led critics to attack it for yet another alleged failing: a head-in-the-sand refusal to become actively involved in social change. The following hypothetical conversation, reprinted from a brochure published by the General Service Board of Alcoholics

Anonymous, shows to what extent AA prizes its independence from the traditional money and power sources that most public services so depend on.

> "Good morning," said the lawyer cheerfully. "I am happy to inform you that under the terms of my late client's will, your fine organization inherits $15,000."
>
> "Sorry," responded the [AA-affiliated] manager just as cheerfully. "We accept no money from anyone except our own members."
>
> "What's the catch?"
>
> "There is no catch. In fact, we won't take more than $500 from our own members in their wills."
>
> After a long pause, the lawyer said: "Oh, I get it. You have so much funding from federal programs that taking contributions would mess up your books."
>
> "As a matter of fact," the manager told him, "in 45 years of existence, we have yet to accept or ask for our first dime from any government—foreign, state, or local."
>
> "Don't you like money?" the lawyer asked incredulously.
>
> "No, we don't," the manager replied. "Our founders believed it wasn't good for us."
>
> "Who told them such a story?" the lawyer asked skeptically.
>
> "Two people: St. Francis of Assisi (whose religious order was based on poverty) and John D. Rockefeller, Jr. (who turned down an early request for money from AA's founders with the sage and oft repeated advice that 'I think money would ruin this.')"

Many more scenarios are featured in AA literature, all reflecting the same recurrent motif: an insistence on remaining independent and uninvolved in public affairs.

Yet there is an irony to the nonaffiliation policy that AA so stubbornly defends. On closer examination, even the most hardened skeptic of self-help is forced to recognize that AA's de facto civil and governmental influence is enormous, even though its de jure policy of nonaffiliation has remained in place like a rock wall for sixty years.

How is it possible to institute societywide changes in the awareness and treatment of high-profile issues like alcoholism and at the same time remain assiduously detached from all forms of activism? The answer provides an interesting lesson in how things are not always what they appear under the big top of power and influence and how a sincerely private, publicity-shy self-help organization can maintain its integrity as a nonaffiliated group and at the same time inspire significant social and legislative changes in the community.

First, individual members of AA became the transmitters of the AA perspective. They carried the message and were in no way limited by AA's nonpolitical dictum. They spread the word out of their commitment; they were not paid publicists.

Second, new forms or institutions, such as the Councils on Alcoholism, were invented to implement the message.

Third, AA's success led to imitation. There are now more than one hundred twelve-step groups modeled after AA. Many of these groups were started by AA members who had other problems as well.

Fourth, committed AA members helped develop new structures such as publishing firms devoted to producing books and pamphlets on every aspect of alcoholism and its treatment.

Fifth, and most recently, a recovering alcoholic organized a direct political arm called the Society of Americans for Recovery (SOAR). Let us take a closer look at how these changes took place.

New Institutions

A significant by-product of the AA movement was the establishment of the government agency called the National Institute on

Alcoholism and Alcohol Abuse. An enormously influential advocate for AA, former Senator Harold Hughes of Iowa, a recovering alcoholic, was the key player in aggressively lobbying for more funding for treatment of alcoholism and an end to discrimination against alcoholics. He introduced the legislation that created the institute. The Hughes Act of 1969–1970 empowered Congress to give large sums of money to states to develop their own alcoholism and drug rehabilitation programs.

Another major structure is the nongovernmental institution known as the National Council on Alcoholism (and its many local councils). Here it was the work of one woman, Marty Mann, coming out of AA, who took on the advocacy role of creating a new structure, a national network of councils to help bring alcoholism into the light. Mann worked tirelessly, traveling the country to set up these centers for alcoholism research, education, and prevention. AA set the stage, and the councils took the mission to the public.

Changes in consciousness and institutional reform are the products of the deep commitment of individual AA members not functioning in an organizational capacity. Their commitment is a product of their firsthand experience with alcoholism and the twelve steps. The individual's experience lends a unique perspective to the creation of new institutions, legislation, and related infrastructure while the parent organization remains free of all this activity.

Although AA disavows social and political action, it does emphasize individual change, and this has led to pervasive institutional changes such as these:

- Acceptance of alcoholism as a disease (by the American Medical Association)

- Application of AA principles in almost all rehabilitation programs for alcohol and drug abuse

- Recommendation by most rehabilitation programs that participants go to Alcoholics Anonymous or Narcotics Anonymous meetings

- Courts' requirement that persons convicted of driving while intoxicated attend AA meetings

- Training programs for certification of alcohol counselors using twelve-step principles

- Employment of recovering alcoholics as personnel in rehabilitation programs

- Development of alcohol councils committed to twelve-step principles

- Founding of publishing companies such as *Hazelden* and magazines such as *Changes* and *Focus* totally committed to twelve-step principles

- Spread of the twelve-step model to over one hundred new groups

- Founding of directly political activist groups such as SOAR

These laws and institutions may not yet have achieved the broad changes in society that political progressives are looking for, but we should not discount these efforts on that ground. These actions play an important role in the politicization of both issues and people. Alcoholism is not the only issue we should be concerned with, but neither should we underestimate the extent to which the AA philosophy may reflect a deep-seated critique of many aspects of life in the United States: excessive individualism, materialism, abuse, the breakdown of human caring, corruption, and so on.

In recent years, a new recovery therapy movement has arisen, powerfully influenced by AA principles, to which large numbers of people are turning for help in dealing with their addictions—alcohol, drugs, gambling, eating, codependency.

Although the therapists practicing this new approach differ in many respects, some major elements stand out:

- Clients are urged to join twelve-step groups offering support from others who have the same or similar histories. These groups, as well as the therapists, call on the individuals to take responsibility for their current behavior.

- Considerable attention is given to exposing and attacking the addictive logic ("stinking thinking") that is characteristic of the participants.

- The therapists often share the same problems as the participants, and this is openly revealed, making the therapeutic process more democratic and symmetrical.

Recovery therapy melds traditional approaches—some borrowed from family systems therapy—with the methodology of the twelve-step movement.

Currently, the twelve-step movement is advancing under the leadership of former Senator Hughes. He remains the guiding spirit behind SOAR, the grassroots political organization group mobilized to end financial, social, legal, and health care discrimination against alcoholics and other drug-dependent people and their families.

Conclusion

Although the self-help approach is often portrayed as individualistic and hence not oriented toward social change, it has actually been in the forefront of social change, most recently manifested in landmark legislation affecting the disabled. An ever-increasing number of self-help groups take strong advocacy stances regarding legislative changes, new rights, and media portrayals. Neighborhood groups are playing a critical role in organizing against drugs and crime.

It is sometimes argued that the social and political action of self-help groups might be focused more sharply—that the interest in the self-help issues deflects from alternative political action. This argument would have more force if there were clear alternatives, well-developed political forms, rather than the deadened, alienated, nonspontaneous political mood of our time. Perhaps a new politics will be born related to the self-help flow—the concern for values that are more than interests, with participatory empowerment as a central motif around issues that are close to people.

In many respects, the self-help movement is giving modern voice to traditional populist themes: cooperation and collective action; empowerment, both individual and social; opposition to bureaucratization; self-determination; emphasis on the informal, the personal, the simple, the direct; a reaffirmation of basic core values related to the role of community, neighborhood, caring, and self-reliance; antielitism and antiexpertism; and a strong antagonism to drugs, hedonism, corruption, and violence. Clearly, the populist cast of the self-help worldview often gives it trouble with modern liberalism. It is noteworthy, however, that the traditionalist bias inherent in much of self-help is counterbalanced by a contemporary emphasis on openness and self-acceptance that has resulted in greater democratization and a demystification of everyday life.

Perhaps in some measure a dialectical tension between a populist and a progressive perspective might be the key to an advanced new politics. We have heard some of the language for this new politics in the speeches of Jesse Jackson, who presents an integration of self-help and progressive political thinking when he calls for a self-reliant, pride-based approach to social change while simultaneously pressing for a broad progressive agenda.

If progressive politicians continue in this direction, we may see a new ideology emerge in which the liberal-conservative continuum has less meaning and self-help philosophy and practice may function to add voices to a platform directed at major social reconstruction.

There is a certain danger in overemphasizing the individual personal change factor—it can be an endpoint in itself; it can divert from social change and become highly individualistic, even narcissistic. But we must recognize that it can also provide commitment and intensity uniting the individual and the community. Self-help has important potential in this context.

Present Limitations and
Future Directions

The central strengths that define self-help are, ironically, also the qualities that set its limits and mark its restrictions. What are these restrictions? And how do they affect the present-day self-help movement?

Problems and Concerns in Today's Self-Help Movement

Relevance of External Help

One limitation derives from the fact that the emphasis in self-help is primarily on positive inner qualities—resourcefulness, independence, the spirit of giving and helping. We have seen this emphasis at work countless times in these pages. At the same time, an intense focus on internal qualities runs the risk of becoming total and thereby exclusionary, shutting out significant *external* factors that may be required to assist in growth.

Certainly, it is useful for a self-help organization to facilitate the inner strengths of its membership and to remain self-reliant. But not to be ignored is the value of outside resources as well—outside knowledge, advice, expertise, and financial support.

In this sense, a neighborhood self-help organization with its focus on sharing, caring, independence, and the group dynamic would be well advised to recognize real benefits and assistance from the outside world and to take advantage of them—help from, say, local clinics, professionals, and state or city agencies.

Trivialization

The high visibility of the self-help movement, its occasional controversiality, and the vulnerability of certain self-help populations all lend themselves to the possibility of trivialization and media exploitation.

Typical is the media coverage of offbeat groups such as victims of alien encounters, clutterers, television addicts, lightning-struck survivors, and the like, at the expense of more representative self-help organizations. For example, the *Wall Street Journal* on October 20, 1992, ran a front-page article headlined "Some Folks Find that Elvis Makes Their Spirits Rise: A Support Group for Psychics Helps the Quick and Dead."

This fascination with exotic and often idiosyncratic self-help populations tends to emphasize the peripheral at the expense of the central, ignoring the major mutual aid organizations that are dedicated to helping people facing serious physical, mental, and social challenges. These organizations include the thousands of groups that administer to the sick, the unemployed, and the disabled and the countless numbers of people concerned with social change, such as Victims for Victims, Self-Help for the Hard of Hearing, the Mental Health Consumers Association, SHARE (for women with breast cancer), SOAR (Society of Americans for Recovery), and hundreds of others concerned with converting the personal into the political.

The process of trivializing self-help was demonstrated in a somewhat different manner via an Oprah Winfrey TV special on the subject of child abuse. Titled *Scared Silent,* this onetime broadcast was deemed so important that in September 1992 it was aired on four channels simultaneously.

Though magnificently produced and frequently touching, not once during the show was mention made of self-help support systems—despite the fact that Winfrey had interviewed countless self-help group members over the years, including many people—parents, children, victims, batterers—directly involved in child abuse cases. Even more frustrating, the recommended follow-up phone numbers flashed on screen at the end of the show failed to provide a single referral to any support group in the country. The entire program, in fact, highlighted professionals, ignoring help organizations such as VOICES (Victims of Incest Can Emerge Survivors), Survivors of Incest Anonymous, SARA (Sexual Assault Recovery Anonymous), Parents Against Molesters, and Parents Anonymous.

The message that emerged from this remarkable media exclusion is clear: compared to professional services, self-help groups are scarcely worth a mention. At best they are novelties suited for curious, sometimes droll cameos on *Oprah*, the *Sally Jesse Raphael Show*, the *Phil Donahue Show*, and other daytime entertainments.

Yet another form of trivialization, perhaps even more insidious than the others, can be found in such anti-self-help books as Wendy Kaminer's *I'm Dysfunctional, You're Dysfunctional* (1992). Kaminer states, for example, that people in self-help recovery groups habitually escape personal accountability for their problems by shifting blame to their parents, thereby making themselves the victims and avoiding the assumption of individual responsibility.

Such a claim is totally at odds with the self-help ethos, whereby people are made to feel responsible for the *solution* to their problem rather than its cause.

For example, supporters of Alcoholics Anonymous take the position that addiction is a disease, the cause of which is beyond the addict's power. But the treatment *is* under the person's control via twelve-step methodology. In this way, the AA disease concept removes the stigma of self-blame and at the same time provides a recovery model based on responsible collective action.

Individual Versus Social Analysis

Critics sometimes point out that empowerment goals in self-help are focused on personal rather than social ends. The self-help movement thus often finds itself tagged as an enterprise that contributes little to social change.

A concomitant critique emanates from the psychologizing and soul searching that may go on during some self-help meetings, reputedly at the expense of social analysis and group action. In part, this approach stems from the belief that the individual is too small and too insignificant to exert an influence on the world at large and that the only place that a person's voice can be heard is in the intimacy of the self-help environment. Such thinking causes people to turn their backs on the larger political institutions that are responsible for establishing actual social policy and real social change.

To these criticisms it is often countered that some self-help groups are in fact political and advocacy-oriented. This is especially true of groups constellated around the women's, gay rights, and disability movements. The fact of the matter is that the self-help modality can be adapted to the needs of introspective groups *or* to advocative organizations that wish to effect national social change. It is this protean, mutable quality that constitutes one of self-help's greatest strengths.

Professionals and Commodification

As social workers, health educators, counselors, and other professionals take an increasingly large role in facilitating support groups and in providing recovery therapy, there is a real danger that the noncommercial, democratic, autonomous, grassroots quality of self-help may be usurped or diluted. Such concerns will become increasingly significant as the self-help community continues to grow.

Organizational Problems

A number of other self-help limitations can be noted. One is that self-help as a movement has little organizational structure. Self-help tends to be multifaceted and to take whatever form is needed at the moment. Indeed, when we speak of self-help, we are in reality speaking of many variations on a theme (mutual aid; self-care; self-help via literature, tapes, and computer programs; professionally facilitated programs), all of which are defined by the needs and circumstances of the moment. This wide range of forms gives self-help breadth and power but at the same time limits its structural integrity and specificity.

Growth itself presents a paradox. As self-help groups increase in number, influence, and exposure; move toward greater participation in advocacy issues; and expand into a more civic arena, the ability to champion a "pure" self-help philosophy (democratic, nonhierarchic, independent, reciprocal, caring) may shrink, the ideals behind it ultimately becoming lost in partisan politics.

In this sense, the expansionary potential of mutual aid may ironically foster a reduction of the self-help principles that originally spawned and nurtured it. It is admittedly difficult to maintain an intimate sharing, caring, self-governing atmosphere when your organization has three million members, as MADD does.

The self-help movement tends to overvalue experiential knowledge and undervalue reflective analysis. Clearly, both experience and reflective thinking should have a place in any complete help system, yet self-help often tends to minimize such elements as scholarship, experiment, theory, systematic controlled analysis, and the scientific method in general. The result is sometimes an imprecise, anecdotal, on-the-fly type of practice that may make loftier claims than available evidence sustains and that remains unsupported by testing, analysis, or hard-core data. "It is so because I experience it that way" goes a certain line of self-help reasoning. At times, the clear air of analysis is necessary to sort things out and put things back on track.

The too-fluid definition of self-help is also a liability. Self-help can seem to be all things to all people. But this can be a complication. After all, how can people make informed decisions or reach valid conclusions when one person is talking about self-help, form A, and another about self-help, form G? Universal definitions are needed. But who is to write them? And is it really possible to cover all elements of this sprawling modality under a single definitional roof? Perhaps answers will emerge as self-help continues to evolve.

A major concern is the possibility that self-help may be used as a substitute for more costly professional services. For example, when dealing with troubled families, it can be dangerous to rely on a mutual aid group in lieu of a caseworker, especially if violence or extreme dysfunctionality is evident.

In general, both interventions should be welcome, caseworker and mutual aid, depending on the circumstances. Commonly, the caseworker may even be called to facilitate development or use of the self-help group.

Future Possibilities in Self-Help

Despite the limitations and uncertainties that self-help groups have faced from the beginning, the self-help movement, with its many styles and models, has clearly proved beneficial to numbers of men, women, and children in a variety of situations. Even relying on narrow research parameters, it is clear that groups have succeeded in providing their membership with a number of social benefits—not to mention the all-important, if less measured, psychological intangibles: a sense of belonging, of making a difference, of self-esteem.

At the same time, however, when seen in relation to the entire American population, the influence of the self-help movement remains relatively untapped.

There are, for example, over ten million widows and two million widowers in the United States, yet only a few thousand groups exist to serve their needs. Over two million senior citizens currently suffer from Alzheimer's disease; a mere handful of mutual aid organizations can be found to help their families and caregivers. Group help is similarly lacking for the millions of people suffering from arthritis, cancer, heart disease, drug addiction, and many other ailments.

Will these unserved populations become more familiar with self-help groups in the future? Will self-help agendas expand into new territory and increase in social importance? Probably. And in the process, professionals will play an increasingly significant role in facilitating self-help.

To accomplish this task in a fully productive way, however, they will require careful training (and retraining), plus an increase in sensitivity to the special needs of such groups (see Chapter Two). Professional education curricula, moreover, will have to give increased attention to the basic principles and philosophy of self-help and to the various ways in which self-help can be successfully applied.

New Models

Combinations of professional-help and self-help systems will likewise have to evolve if physical and mental health populations are to be fully served. New models will be called for, many of which we have described elsewhere in this book (especially in Chapters Four and Six)—recall the case in which mental health consumers provided mental health services to other patients or the reciprocal tutoring programs and peer helpers in elementary and secondary schools.

At the core of these new models, as we have seen, lies the fundamental self-help principle of converting needs and problems into assets. One of the backbone supports of the mutual aid movement, this concept is based on employing the skills and experience of people who have successfully coped with certain problems (recovery, disease, disability) to help others overcome the same difficulties. Later on, helpees return this favor by helping still others in a continuous chain of need and reciprocity.

In this way, resources are continually grown and nurtured within the help environment itself. The growth and resource exploitation process turns on its own pivot in a state of perpetual helping motion.

Increasing Politicization

We are also likely to see an awareness of self-help philosophy expand in the national political consciousness. For this to occur successfully, there must be a transfer of the positive skills and attitudes acquired in self-help activity into the larger bailiwick of the state and government.

Many inroads have, of course, already been made in this direction. The antismoking movement, which began in small "smoke stoppers" groups, is today widely politicized and largely responsible for the passage of sweeping antismoking legislation. The gay rights movement, which started, both metaphorically and literally, in rooms with blinds drawn, is today a conspicuous political force.

Increased Unification

We are also apt to see an increasing unification of the self-help movement, along with a reduction of its fragmentation and compartmentalization. To expedite this transition, a "national alliance for self-help" or some such institution may soon appear, with a cross-country network similar to the national hookup developed by the disability rights movement.

Building toward this objective, an increased role is anticipated for advocacy self-help groups and coalitions. Related trends along these lines are already clear:

- A considerable expansion of electronic self-help facilities is expected in the United States via such on-line resources as CompuServe and the Internet. Disabled people, especially shut-ins, stand to benefit greatly from such aids. (It is both ironic and significant that the credo of the Internet, as stated in Steven Levy's 1984 book *Hackers*, features axioms such as "Access to computers should be unlimited and total," "All information should be free," and "Mistrust authority and promote decentralization," which, mutatis mutandis, could be lines from a self-help credo as well.)

- Conflict management programs, specifically ones that feature self-help paradigms, will multiply in our schools, where violence is common.

- As unemployment rates continue to be high (even in an improving economy), self-help groups for the unemployed will increase commensurately.

- Consensus is likely to grow among self-help group members that accepting aid and resources from the government does not necessarily compromise a group's integrity. We may also see increasing involvement of the government in the self-help movement in general.

- The twelve-step movement will continue to expand and will begin to administer to a wide spectrum of chronic illnesses, including cancer, multiple sclerosis, and heart disease.

- A great deal more research and testing will be generated in the academic and social science communities sampling the effectiveness of the self-help approach (or lack thereof). The data obtained from these studies will provide a clearer picture of self-help's strengths and weaknesses.

Productivity: A New Direction for Self-Help

If we read the present signs correctly, the use of self-help principles to increase productivity in public agencies may soon become a trend.

Case in point: it is acknowledged that education, experience, and motivation are powerful factors for increasing productivity. The self-help consumer is likely to generate all three of these attributes in an almost automatic way. For example, self-help consumers have experiential knowledge related to the service consumed and are highly motivated by the fact that this knowledge concerns their own particular problems and needs.

The rape victim, the widow, the spina bifida patient, and the parents of murdered children all possess specialized knowledge born of experience that uniquely qualifies them to provide specifically tailored helping services to others suffering from the same problem—and hence to boost the productive helping output of the public or private agency involved.

The consumer-as-producer phenomenon aids human productivity in countless ways, especially in the field of human services. Studies show that self-care practices such as taking one's own blood pressure or administering one's own insulin are highly effective techniques that add to the productivity of the health system. They also free doctors to perform more urgent and more demanding tasks. ·

Hospital- and clinic-based self-help groups (such as cancer support groups) have increased patients' longevity and quality of life. This service boosts the productivity of presiding agencies and of the professionals involved in facilitating these groups.

Tenant management of public housing complexes has been found to reduce crime and property destruction dramatically. Tenant management groups therefore contribute direct benefits to the productivity of state and local housing agencies and police. The reduction in neighborhood vandalism reduces expenditures for municipal agencies and private citizens alike.

Neighborhood anticrime groups throughout the country, working in conjunction with local police, are reported to have reduced crime in many areas, thereby increasing law enforcement productivity and relieving some of the burden of local police departments.

Peer tutoring in schools has proved to be a highly effective intervention using self-help principles (reciprocal aid, helpee as helper, consumer as producer) and can increase the productivity of the school system in general.

And a one-on-one peer approach among young contemporaries has proved to be an effective intervention for reducing drug abuse, increasing the productivity of the counseling staff.

In each of these examples—and there are many more—the self-help approach adds to the productivity of individual agencies and the commonwealth at large. A prime example is found in the use of AA's twelve-step methodology. As we have seen, research data for this approach do not provide conclusive answers as to whether AA's methods are necessarily better than those of other antialcohol interventions. However, the fact that AA's methodology discourages alcohol abuse among participants and hence reduces absenteeism and layoffs in the workplace (along with accidents, drinking-related health problems, medical insurance payouts, early burnout, and worker inefficiency) makes it clear that its contributions to the conservation of society's economic resources are considerable.

Empowerment and Threats to Empowerment

Consumer involvement in the expansion of productivity is, in many cases, personally empowering as well as collectively productive. Instead of remaining dependent clients, consumers become active participants in the ongoing affairs of their own lives and the lives of others.

This bit of bull-by-the-horns activism not only improves the quantity of services produced—motivated people work more efficiently than indifferent people—but enhances the quality as well. A neighborhood where citizens pitch in to reduce littering is vastly different from a neighborhood where residents fling wrappers and beer cans into the gutter. The difference is not just one of appearances; it speaks of intangibles, of pride and community spirit. A housing project that is managed by its tenants is a vastly different living environment than one in which tenants have no say. The climate in a school where students tutor and counsel one another is qualitatively different from the traditional teacher-centered, competition-driven classroom and hence a good deal more effective at encouraging students to learn.

In the cases cited here, and many more like them, there appears to be a convergence of interests among all parties concerned. One of the dangers to be aware of in such circumstances, however, is that the objectives of human service providers are at times inconsistent with—or, in the worst case, in opposition to—those of the consumers receiving their services.

If, let us say for the sake of argument, the Department of Health and Human Services were to involve its client consumers more fully in education programs, would this be done to help welfare recipients function more effectively while receiving benefits? Or would it be directed toward removing clients from the welfare rolls entirely? In such cases, it is not always certain that the goals of the agency and the goals of the consumer are congruent.

A study done in Atlanta revealed that peer counseling was a highly effective tool for encouraging sexual abstinence among eighth graders and that the rate of sexually transmitted diseases dropped commensurately when it was used. The result is admirable, but what is potentially troubling here is the imposing of a moral message that may or may not be acceptable to everyone concerned, one that in certain ways curtails individual freedom of choice.

Even more troubling is the possibility of direct government involvement in the sphere of self-help. The prospect of federal agencies regulating self-help curricula or forcing group leaders to obtain state licensing credentials threatens to subvert the freedom and autonomy that the movement was founded on.

Only the self-help ethos itself, with its emphasis on empowerment and self-determination, stands in the way of such dangers. Indeed, the strength and durability of the movement lie ultimately not in its form or organization but in its values, spirit, resilience, and ability to remain autonomous.

Though a great deal more research is needed concerning the effectiveness of self-help methods, we believe that there is considerable social support for increased utilization of the self-help paradigm.

This book has emphasized the mutual aid form of help, including professionally facilitated self-help groups and, to a lesser extent, the expression of self-help ideas through peer help and consumer-managed mental health services. Other forms of self-help will also bear study, of course, and certainly there is a pressing need for further investigation of such related areas as self-help literature (bibliotherapy), alternative forms and structures of self-help, and the productivity involved in such promising quasi-self-help projects as community law enforcement, tenant-managed public housing, and probationary services.

The potential power of self-help rests on its basic principles:

- Self-determination

- Decommodification and freely donated services

- A democratic philosophy exemplified in rotating group leadership, nonhierarchic structure, and the acceptance of troubled, stigmatized behavior

- Emphasis on the importance of experiential learning

- The struggle against expertism, mystification, exclusivity, elitism, and professional privatization of knowledge (as demonstrated most clearly in self-help's democratizing of patient populations and in the promotion of medical self-care and patients' rights)

Yet even though research has borne out the effectiveness of self-help activities (including self-help books, literature, and tapes), self-help strategies have so far been applied to only a fraction of the help-seeking populations. There are several reasons for this.

Despite the healing power of inner resources, many problems addressed by self-help groups also require significant external and professional attention. This attention is often unavailable to self-help groups and is sometimes shunned by them.

The fact remains, however, that professionals are becoming involved in self-help activities at an increasing rate; to deny this trend is to deny reality and the wave of the future as well. It is noteworthy that David Spiegel (1993), whose highly successful work in extending the life (and improving the quality of life) of cancer patients conspicuously combines self-help principles (such as the helper therapy principle) with professionally based services and professional leadership.

Also, except for such time-tested organizations as Alcoholic Anonymous, many contemporary self-help groups have not yet found their ideal structure. This means that self-help techniques are often limited to a single intervention mode that does not fully address the needs of all its potential clients.

Witness, for example, violence in the schools. It may well be that school-based peer approaches will someday exert an impact on the American school system as great as AA's on alcoholism. For such ends to be achieved, however, a single approach, such as peer mediation, valuable as it is, cannot remain the primary centerpiece in the educational process. It must be buttressed by supplementary methods (as described in Chapter Six) such as reciprocal learning, cooperative learning, peer mentoring, and peer mutual aid of all types, all of which are ultimately directed toward changing the school ethos and to shifting power to the student constituency—in short, the creation of a peer-centered school.

The fragmentary, disunified nature of the self-help movement is expressed not merely by the fact that it addresses a wide spectrum of problem situations but also by its diverse and not always complementary forms (self-care, mutual aid, peer helping, twelve-step plans, non-twelve-step plans, professionally facilitated groups, non-professionally facilitated groups, and so forth). If fragmentation is reduced but the vital elements of self-help are left intact, results similar to those gained by such successful groups as the disabled rights movement may be achieved. The aim is to develop a series of self-help models that effectively transform helpees into helpers. These models can then be applied to large segments of the population and will go a long way toward bringing aid to millions of unserved men, women, and children across the country.

In the future, therefore, it is hoped that these and many other related issues will be addressed specifically in the context of the ideas that have been proposed throughout this book: namely, a new pathway to social productivity via self-help, one that embodies the principles of the consumer as producer, the conversion of problems into assets, the expansion of resources from within, the interchangeability of helper and helpee roles, a positive ethos, emphasis on direct experience, and a democratic structure. This will ultimately provide better services for society, encourage community solidarity, and produce more fully empowered, more effective citizens.

Notes

· ·

Chapter One

1. Mutual aid can nevertheless be regarded as a form of self-help in contrast to group therapy, which features a formal leader and a professionally based system of thought arising from outside the group. This is true even in cases where the particular system of group therapy may emphasize the need for the involvement of the group at the deepest level. This involvement is always framed by the external therapist and his or her system of therapy.

2. The effects of external assistance can vary greatly, ranging from efforts to draw out internal motion or responsiveness to dictatorial imposition ("Do it this way," "That is how you do it").

3. To grasp this, we must jetisson the old distinction formerly made between individual help and group mutual aid.

4. A popular usage of the term *addiction* applies it to any intense involvement—for example, being "addicted" to running or watching football. Such things may be rare examples of complex addictions, but mere intense involvement does not meet the formal definition.

5. It is quite possible, of course, that the second type of drinker can become attracted to AA (as the only game in town) and benefit from an intervention that in some ways is more than they need. This may be essentially harmless, but the intensity of AA amounts to overkill—it forces them to identify as alcoholics, admit to having

a disease, and center much of their lives around an unnecessary intervention strategy.

6. Modern narcissism does not stem from inner love but rather from an emptiness that is constantly fed by innovative external products and processes loaded with promises and short-run mood manipulators that provide distraction, temporary reduction of tensions, and a lifetime of seduction.

7. Implicit in this formulation is a dialectic, an opposition of the inner and outer dimensions but also a unity—both inner and outer forms of help are necessary (the unity and the struggle of opposites).

Chapter Two

1. For a full discussion of present-day professionals, see Charles Derber and others (1990). See especially pages 12–18, all of Chapter Twelve, and the "postscript" on pages 211–227 for a valuable review of major positions on professionalism, including those of Alvin W. Gouldner, Eliot Freidson, Barbara and John Ehrenreich, and Daniel Bell.

Chapter Three

1. If the self-selection process is efficient, it may be that most of this group represents AA's true alcoholic—or at least seriously addicted—population. Many persons who drop out of AA or have alcohol dependencies of a general kind may in fact benefit from other interventions. Some of them may even recover without outside assistance.

2. The problem with the concept of serenity prayer is that at any point in time it may be true that I cannot change A, and if I don't accept that, I will be hitting my head against a brick wall; but the situation needs to be checked very carefully because new approaches, new technology, or new knowledge may enable me to change what seemed unchangeable, and perhaps I won't know unless I try harder. The effort to test limits may be significant in producing a change.

And there is always a danger of a negative self-fulfilling prophecy—
I believe that the situation cannot be changed and act accordingly,
thereby reinforcing the status quo.

3. Some clarification is needed. The *recovery movement* encompasses
recovery that may take place in twelve-step groups, as well as in
professionally led recovery therapy and rehabilitation centers, in-
patient programs, and the like. *Recovery therapy* refers to professionally led treatment based on twelve-step principles but delivered by
psychologists, social workers, and other trained professionals.
Unlike the recovery that takes place in twelve-step groups, this
treatment is not free of charge.

Chapter Eight

1. See Chesler (1991) for a review of social advocacy efforts made by
self-help groups, particularly oriented toward changing professional
and bureaucratic behaviors.

References

Albee, G. "An Ounce of Prevention: Reorienting Mental Health Priorities." *Self-Help Reporter*, 1981, *5*, 1–2.

"Alternative Medicine: The Facts." *Consumer Reports*, Jan. 1994, pp. 51–53.

Benard, B. *The Case for Peers*. Portland, Ore.: Far West Laboratory for Educational Research and Development, 1990.

Bloom, B. S. "The Search for Methods as Effective as One-on-One Tutoring." *Educational Leadership*, 1984, *41*(8), 4–7.

Blume, S. "Gambling: Disease or 'Excuse'? High Rollers Suffer from an Illness." *U.S. Journal of Drug and Alcohol Dependence*, August 1989, pp. 73–77.

Borkman, T. "Experiential Knowledge: A New Conception for the Analysis of Self-Help Groups." *Health and Social Work*, 1976, *10*, 95–103.

Boston Women's Health Book Collective. *Our Bodies, Ourselves*. New York: Simon & Schuster, 1976.

Brint, S. *In an Age of Experts: The Changing Role of Professionals in Politics and Public Life*. Princeton, N.J.: Princeton University Press, 1994.

Budd, S., and Harp, H. "Suggestions for Consumer-Run Programs." *The Self-Helper*, July 1991, pp. 4–5.

Cardinal, J., and Farquharson, A. *The Self-Help Resource Kit: Training Materials to Enhance Professional Support of Self-Help Groups*. Victoria, B.C.: University of Victoria, 1991.

Carnes, P. *Out of the Shadows: Understanding Sexual Addiction*. Minneapolis: CompCare, 1983.

Cary, R. G. "The Widowed: A Year Later." *Journal of Consulting Psychology*, 1977, *24*, 125–131.

Chamberlin, J. *On Our Own: Patient-Controlled Alternatives to the Mental Health System*. New York: McGraw-Hill, 1978.

Chesler, M. "Mobilizing Consumer Activism in Health Care: The Role of Self-Help Groups." In M. Chesler, *Research in Social Movements, Conflicts and Change*. Greenwich, Conn.: JAI Press, 1991.

Clayton, P. J. "Mortality and Morbidity in the First Year of Bereavement." *Archives of General Psychiatry*, 1974, *30*, 747–750.

Cloward, R. "Teenagers as Tutors of Academically Low-Achieving Children: Impact on Tutors and Tutees." In V. L. Allen (ed.), *Children as Teachers*. San Diego, Calif.: Academic Press, 1976.

Cohen, P. A., and others. "Educational Outcomes of Peer Tutoring: A Metanalysis of Findings." *American Educational Research Journal*, 1982, *19*(2), 237–248.

Damon, W., and Phelps, E. "Strategic Users of Peer Learning in Children's Education." In T. Berndt and G. Ladd (eds.), *Peer Relationships in Child Development*. New York: Wiley, 1989.

Derber, C., Schwartz, W. A., and Magrass, Y. *Power in the Highest Degree: Professionals and the Rise of a New Mandarin Order*. New York: Oxford University Press, 1990.

Dewar, T. "Professionalized Clients as Self-Helpers." In *Self-Help and Health: A Report*. New York: New Human Service Institute, Queens College, City University of New York, 1976.

Dorsman, J. *How to Quit Drinking Without AA: A Complete Self-Help Guide*. Rocklin, Calif.: Prima, 1994.

Dory, F., and Riessman, F. "Training Professionals in Organizing Self-Help Groups." *Citizen Participation*, Jan.-Feb. 1982, pp. 7–9.

Du Pont, R. L., and McGovern, J. P. *A Bridge to Recovery: An Introduction to Twelve-Step Programs*. Washington, D.C.: American Psychiatric Press, 1994.

Eisenberg, D. M., Kessler, R., and Foster, C. "Unconventional Medicine in the United States: Prevalence, Costs, and Patterns of Use." *New England Journal of Medicine*, 1993, *328*, 246–252.

Emerick, R. "Group Demographics in the Mental Patient Movement: Group Location, Age, and Size as Structural Factors." *Community Mental Health Journal*, 1989, *25*(4), 277–380.

Emerick, R. "The Politics of Psychiatric Self-Help: Political Factions, Interactional Support, and Group Longevity in a Social Movement." *Social Science and Medicine*, 1991, *32*(10), 1122–1128.

Fisher, J. D., Nadler, A., and Whitcher-Alagna, S. "Recipient Reactions to Aid." *Psychological Bulletin*, 1982, *92*(1), 27–54.

Foa, F. C., and Foa, E. B. "Resource Exchange: Toward a Structured Theory of Interpersonal Communication." In A. W. Siegman and B. Pope (eds.), *Studies in Dyadic Communication*. Elmsford, N.Y.: Pergamon Press, 1971.

Forbes, D. *False Fixes: The Cultural Policies of Drugs, Alcohol, and Addictive Relations*. Albany: State University Press of New York, 1994.

Fromm, E. *Man for Himself: An Inquiry into the Psychology of Ethics*. Austin, Texas: Holt, Rinehart and Winston, 1947.

Fuchs, V. "Health Care and the United States Economic System." *Millbank Memorial Quarterly*, 1972, *50*(2), 16–22.

Galanter, M. "Zealous Self-Help Groups as an Adjunct to Psychiatric Treatment: A Study of Recovery." *American Journal of Psychiatry*, 1988, *145*, 1248–1253.

Gartner, A., and Riessman, F. *The Service Society and the Consumer Vanguard*. New York: HarperCollins, 1974.

Gartner, A. J. "A Typology of Women's Self-Help Groups." *Social Policy*, 1985, *15*(4), 25–30.

Gartner, A. J., and Riessman, F. "Peer Tutoring: Toward a New Model." *ERIC Digest*, 1993, *93*(2), 1–4.

Glassman, A. "Cigarette Smoking: Implications for Psychiatric Illness." *American Journal of Psychiatry*, 1993, *150*, 546–553.

Glover, R. W., and Steber, S. From the Back Wards to the Boardroom: The Empowerment of Mental Health Consumers. Unpublished paper, University of Michigan, November 1989.

Goodman, G., and Jacobs, M. "The Self-Help, Mutual-Support Group." In A. Fuhriman and G. Burlingame (eds.), *Handbook of Group Psychology*. New York: Wiley, 1994.

Gordon, R. D., and others. "Factors in Postpartum Emotional Adjustment." *Obstetrical Gynecology*, 1965, *25*, 156–166.

Gordon, R. E., and others. "Reducing Hospitalization of State Mental Patients: Peer Management and Support." In A. Yaeger and R. Slotkin (eds.), *Community Mental Health*. New York: Plenum, 1982.

Gouldner, A. W. "The Norm of Reciprocity: A Preliminary Statement." *American Sociological Review*, 1960, *25*, 161–179.

Greenwood, C. R., and others. "Longitudinal Effects of Classwide Peer Tutoring" *Journal of Educational Psychology*, 1989, *81*(3), 371–383.

Harvard Mental Health Letter, Aug. 1992.

Harvard Mental Health Letter, Mar.-Apr. 1993.

Hassen, S. *Combating Cults*. Rochester, NY: Park Street Press, 1988.

Hazelden News & Professional Update, July 1994, pp. 1–3.

Hedin, D. "Students as Teachers: A Tool for Improving School Climate and Productivity." *Social Policy*, 1987, *17*(3), 42–47.

Hinrichsen, G., Revenson, T., and Shinn, M. "Does Self-Help Help? An Empirical Investigation of Scoliosis Peer Support Groups." *Journal of Social Issues*, 1985, *41*(1), 65–87.

Holden, L. "The Man Who Eradicated Polio—30 Years Later: Jonas Salk." *Continental*, Mar. 1985, p. 70.

Ho, M. K., and Norlin, J. "The Helper Therapy Principle and the Creation of a Therapeutic Milieu." *Child Care Quarterly*, 1974, *3*, 109–118.

Jensen, P. S. "Risk, Protective Factors, and Supportive Interventions in Chronic Airway Obstruction." *Archives of General Psychiatry*, 1983, *40*(11), 70–74.

Johnson, R., and Johnson, D. "The Socialization and Achievement Crisis: Are Cooperative Learning Experiences the Solution?" In *Applied Social Psychology Annual 4*. New York: Sage, 1983.

Kallman, B. J. "Are You Aware?" *Let's Live*, Jan. 1994, pp. 17–25.

Kaminer, W. *I'm Dysfunctional, You're Dysfunctional*. Reading, Mass.: Addison-Wesley, 1992.

Kasl, C. D. *Many Roads, One Journey: Moving Beyond the Twelve Steps*. New York: HarperPerennial, 1992.

Katz, A. *Partners in Wellness: Self-Help Groups and Professionals*. Sacramento: California Department of Mental Health, Office of Prevention, 1987.

Katz, A. *Self-Help in America: A Social Movement Perspective*. New York: Twayne, 1993.

Katz, A., and Bender, E. *The Strength in Us: Self-Help Groups in the Modern World*. New York: New Viewpoints, 1976.

Kaufman, C. "Roles for Mental Health Consumers in Self-Help Group Research." *Journal of Applied Behavioral Science*, 1993, *29*(2), 257–271.

Kelly, H. J. "The Effect of the Helping Experience upon the Self-Concept of the Helper." Unpublished doctoral dissertation, University of Pittsburgh, 1973.

King, B. T., and Janis, I. L. "Comparison of the Effectiveness of Improvised Responses Versus Role Playing Producing Opinion Changes." *Human Relations*, 1956, *1*, 177–186.

Kurtz, E., and Ketcham, K. *The Spirituality of Imperfection*. New York: Bantam Books, 1992.

Kurtz, L. F. "The Self-Help Movement: Review of the Past Decade of Research." *Social Work with Groups*, 1990, *13*(3), 23–40.

Levin, H., Glass, G., and Weister, G. *Cost Effectiveness of Four Educational Interventions*. Project Report No. 84. Stanford, Calif.: Stanford University, 1984.

Levin, L., Katz, A., and Holtz, E. *Self-Care: Lay Initiatives in Health*. New York: Prodist, 1976.

Levy, L. "Issues in Research and Evaluation." In A. J. Gartner and F. Riessman (eds.), *The Self-Help Revolution*. New York: Human Sciences Press, 1984.

Levy, S. *Hackers: Heroes of the Computer Revolution*. Garden City, NY: Anchor Press/Doubleday, 1984.

Lieberman, M. A. "Self-Help Groups and Psychiatry." *American Psychiatric Association Annual Review*, 1986, *5*, 744–760.

Lieberman, M. A., and Borman, L. D. "The Impact of Self-Help Groups on Widows' Mental Health." *National Reporter*, 1991, *4*, 2–6.

Lieberman, M. A., and Snowden, L. R. "Problems in Assessing Prevalence and Membership Characteristics of Self-Help Group Participants." *Journal of Applied Behavioral Science*, 1993, *29*(2), 166–180.

Low, A. *Mutual Health Through Will Training: A System of Self-Help in Psychotherapy as Practiced by Recovery, Inc.* Boston: Christopher, 1971.

Luks, A. *The Helping Power of Doing Good: The Health and Spiritual Benefits of Helping Others*. New York: Fawcett Columbine, 1991.

Madara, E., and White B. (eds.). *The Self-Help Sourcebook*. Denville, N.J.: St. Claire's–Riverside Medical Center, 1992.

Maddison, D. C., and Viola, A. "The Health of Widows in the Year Following Bereavement." *Journal of Psychiatry*, 1964, *110*, 198–204.

Marris, P. *Widows and Their Families*. London: Routledge, 1958.

Maxwell, M. A. *The AA Experience*. New York: McGraw-Hill, 1984.

Medvene, L. Selected Highlights of Research on Effectiveness of Self-Help Groups. Unpublished paper, California Self-Help Center, Los Angeles, 1990.

Member's-Eye View of Alcoholics Anonymous, A. New York: Alcoholics Anonymous World Services, 1970.

Milam, J. "The Alcoholism Revolution." *Professional Counselor*, Aug. 1992, pp. 15–30.

Milam, J., and Ketcham, K. *Under the Influence*. New York: Bantam Books, 1981.

Mundis, J. *How to Get Out of Debt, Stay Out of Debt, and Live Prosperously*. New York: Bantam Books, 1990.

Osborne, D., and Gaebler, T. *Reinventing Government: How the Entrepreneurial Spirit Is Transforming the Public Sector from Schoolhouse to Statehouse, City Hall to Pentagon*. Reading, Mass.: Addison-Wesley, 1992.

Parkes, C. M. "Recent Bereavement as a Cause of Mental Illness." *British Journal of Psychiatry*, 1964, *110*, 198–204.

Parkes, C. M. *Bereavement: Studies of Grief in Adult Life*. London: Tavistock, 1972.

Pearl, A., and Riessman, F. *New Careers for the Poor: The Nonprofessional in Human Services*. New York: Free Press, 1965.

Peele, S. *The Diseasing of America: Addiction Treatment Out of Control*. Lexington, Mass.: Lexington Books, 1989.

Peele, S., and Brodsky, A. *The Truth About Addiction and Recovery*. New York: Simon & Schuster, 1991.

Powell, T. J., "Self-Help Research and Policy Issues." *Journal of Applied Behavioral Sciences*, 1993, *29*(2), 151–165.

Prochaska, J., and others. "In Search of How People Change: Applications to Addictive Behaviors." *American Psychologist*, 1992, *47*, 1102–1114.

Raiff, N. "Some Health-Related Outcomes of Self-Help Participation: Recovery, Inc., as a Case Example of a Self-Help Organization in Mental Health." In A. Gartner and F. Riessman (eds.), *The Self-Help Revolution*. New York: Human Sciences Press, 1984.

Rappaport, J., and others. "Collaborative Research with a Mutual Help Organization." *Social Policy*, 1985, *15*(3), 12–24.

Richardson, J. "Determinants of Adjustment to Laryngectomy Surgery." Unpublished doctoral dissertation, School of Public Health, University of California, Los Angeles, 1980.

Roberts, L. "Giving and Receiving Help: Group Behavioral Predictors of Outcomes for Members of a Mutual Help Organization." Unpublished doctoral dissertation, University of Illinois, Urbana, 1989.

"Rx: Helping Others." *Mind/Body Health Newsletter*, Winter 1993, p. 3. (Published by the Center for Health Sciences/Institute for the Study of Human Knowledge, Los Altos, Calif.)

Schaef, A. W. *When Society Becomes an Addict*. San Francisco: HarperCollins, 1987.

Schaef, A. W., and Fassel, D. *The Addictive Organization*. San Francisco: HarperCollins, 1988.

Shearn, M. A., and Fireman, B. H. "Stress Management and Mutual Support Groups in Rheumatoid Arthritis." *American Journal of Medicine*, 1985, *78*(5), 23–27.

Shroeder, D. A., and others. *The Social Psychology of Helping and Altruism: Problems and Puzzles*. New York: McGraw-Hill, in press.

Sidel, R., and Sidel, V. "Beyond Coping." *Social Policy*, 1976, *7*(2), 67–69.

Silverman, P. R. *Widow to Widow*. New York: Springer, 1986.

Skovholt, T. M. "The Client as Helper: A Means to Promote Psychological Growth." *Counseling Psychologist*, 1974, *4*, 58–64.

Social Policy, 1987, *18*(2), cover.

Spiegel, D. *Living Beyond Limits: New Hope and Help for Facing Life-Threatening Illness*. New York: New York Times Books, 1993.

Stewart, M. "Expanding Theoretical Conceptualizations of Self-Help Groups." *Social Science and Medicine*, 1990, *31*(9), 1057–1066.

Strauss, A. "Chronic Illness." *Society*, 1973, *10*, 26–36.

Swengel, E. M. "Peer Tutoring: Back to the Roots of Peer Helping." *Peer Facilitator Quarterly*, 1991, *8*(4), 28–32.

Swift, C. "The Prevention Equation and Self-Help Groups." *Self-Help Reporter*, 1979, *3*(4), 1–2.

Tobler, N. "Metanalysis of 143 Adolescent Drug Prevention Problems: Quantitative Outcome Results of Program Participants Compared to a Control or Comparison Group." *Journal of Drug Issues*, 1986, *16*, 537–567.

Toffler, A. *The Third Wave*. New York: Morrow, 1980.

Toseland, R. W., Rossiter, C. M., and Labreque, M. S. "The Effectiveness of Two Kinds of Support Groups for Caregivers." *Social Service Review*, 1989, *63*, 415–432.

Upledger, J. E. "Self-Discovery and Self-Healing." In R. Carlson and B. Shield (eds.), *Healers on Healing*. Los Angeles: Tarcher, 1989.

U.S. Department of Health and Human Services. *Surgeon General's Workshop on Self-Help and Public Health*. Washington, D.C.: U.S. Government Printing Office, 1987.

Vachon, M.L.S., and others. "A Controlled Study of Self-Help Intervention for Widows." *American Journal of Psychiatry*, 1980, *137*, 1380–1384.

Vaillant, G. E. *The Natural History of Alcoholism*. Cambridge, Mass.: Harvard University Press, 1983.

Van Rooijen, L. "Widow's Bereavement: Stress and Depression After 1.5 Years." In I. Sarason (ed.), *Stress and Anxiety*. New York: Wiley, 1981.

Videcka-Sherman, L., and Leiberman, M. A. "The Effects of Self-Help and Psychotherapy Intervention on Child Loss: The Limits of Recovery." *American Journal of Orthopsychiatry*, 1985, *55*, 70–82.

Weiner, M. F., and Caldwell, T. "The Process and Impact of an ICU Nurse Support Group." *International Journal of Psychiatry in Medicine*, 1983–84, *13*(1), 63–80.

Weiss, R. S. "The Contributions of an Organization of Single Parents to the Well-Being of Its Members." *Family Coordinator*, 1973, *22*, 321–326.

Wilson, B. *Alcoholics Anonymous*. New York: Works Publishing, 1939.

Wollert, R., and others. "Help Giving in Behavioral Control and Stress-Coping Self-Help Groups." *Small Group Behavior*, 1982, *13*, 52–70.

Zinman, S., Harp, H., and Budd, S. (eds.). *Reaching Across: Mental Health Clients Helping Each Other*. Sacramento, Calif.: California Network of Mental Health Clients, 1987.

Index